The Miles Color Atlas of
Infectious Diseases

Second Edition

R. T. D. Emond

MB, ChB (St And), FRCP (Lond), DTM & H (Eng)
Consultant Physician, Infectious Diseases Department,
The Royal Free Hospital, London,
Honorary Associate Physician,
Hospital for Tropical Diseases, London,
Honorary Senior Lecturer, University of London

H. A. K. Rowland

MA, DM, PhD, FRCP, DTM & H
Department of Clinical Tropical Medicine,
London School of Hygiene and Tropical Medicine, London

MILES

Copyright © R.T.D. Emond, 1974, 1987
Copyright © R.T.D. Emond and H.A.K. Rowland, 1987
Second edition published by Wolfe Medical Publications Ltd, 1987

ISBN 0 7234 0973 0 cased edition
ISBN 0 7234 0957 9 limp edition

General Editor, Wolfe Medical Atlases: G. Barry Carruthers,
MD(London)

Printed by Hazell Books, Aylesbury, Bucks., England
Member of BPCC Ltd.

This book is one of the titles in the series of Wolfe Medical
Atlases, a series that brings together probably the world's
largest systematic published collection of diagnostic
colour photographs.
This edition is published for Miles Inc., Pharmaceutical Division
by Wolfe Publishing, London, U.K. in association with:
Caduceus Medical Publishers Inc.
Patterson, NY, USA.

ACKNOWLEDGEMENTS

It would have been impossible to illustrate so many aspects of infection without the generosity and support of numerous friends and colleagues, who have provided photographs from their collections. We are most grateful to them for the following illustrations:

Dr June Almeida, **336**; Dr Isobel Beswick, **39**; Professor C.P. Beattie, Professor J.K.A. Beverley and the Department of Photography, The United Sheffield Hospitals, **442–4**, **446**, **448–9**; Dr A. Bloom, **41** and **57**; Dr Jean Bradley, **9**, **10**, **45–7**, **67**, **92–3**, **124**, **137**, **452**; the late Dr R.T. Brain, **293**; the late Dr E.H. Brown, **130**, **138**, **260**, **329**; Dr G. Laing Brown, **223–4**; Dr A.D.M. Bryceson, **150**, **153**; Dr D.C. MacDonald Burns, **201**; Dr K.C. Carstairs and the editor of the *Proceedings of the Royal Society of Medicine*, **229–30**; Dr L.S. Carstairs, **225–8**; Dr A.B. Christie, **231**, **407**; Mr C. Daniels, **411**; Professor S. Darougar, **184–5**; Mr D. Downton, **139**; Professor J.A. Dudgeon and the Hospital for Sick Children, London, who retain the copyright, **360–1**, **371**, **373**, **376**; Dr A.J. Duggan, **173**; Professor K.R. Dumbell, **268–9**; Dr G.J. Ebrahim, **437**; Dr Anne M. Field and Mr A. Porter, **205**, **311**, **320**, **378**, **404**; Dr W.J.D. Fleming, **299**; Dr T.H. Flewett, **112**; Dr J.A. Forbes, **160**; Dr W. Frain-Bell and the Department of Dermatology, University of Dundee, **50**, **419–20**; Dr G.A. Gresham, **163**, **415**, **453**; Mr N.D.F. Grindley, **91**; Dr S. Haider, **284**; Dr K.K. Hussain, **109**; Dr W.M. Jamieson, **20**, **87**, **131**, **133**, **165**, **343**, **405–6**, **408–10**, **418**; Mr J.J. Kanski, **181**; Dr T. Kawasaki, **470–5**, **477–8**; Dr S.G. Lamb, **15**, **34**, **210**, **251**, **286**, **300**, **355**, **447**, **465**; Professor H.P. Lambert, **377**, **450–1**; Dr J.H. Lawson, **171**; Dr J.J. Linehan, **344**, **352**, **368**; Dr S. Lucas, **147–8**, **431**, **440–1**; Dr J. Luder, **73**, **356**; Mrs S.D. Marston, **298**; Dr J.M. Medlock, **17–19**, **42**, **52**, **126**, **158**, **381**; Mr I. McCaul, **58**; Dr G.D.W. McKendrick, **60**, **78**, **159**, **199**; Dr W.F.T. McMath, Dr K.K. Hussain and the Editor and publisher of the *British Medical Journal*, **485–6**; Dr E. Montuschi, **84**; Dr J.McC. Murdoch and Dr J.A. Gray, **29** and **53**; Dr R.O. Murray, **107–8**, **110**; Professor I.C.S. Normand, **370**; Dr R.J. Olds, **48**, **85**, **121**, **123**, **125**, **141**, **157**, **168**; the late Dr E.P. O'Sullivan, **55**, **56**, **86**, **88**, **215**, **359**, **374**, **393**; Dr G. Pampiglione, **358**; Dr J.D.J. Parker, **290–1**; Dr H.G. Prentice, **297**; Dr J.I. Pugh, **272–3**, **277**, **487**; Dr C.S. Ratnatunga, **188**, **200**; Dr G.H. Ree, **203–4**; Dr D. Taylor-Robinson, **206–7**; Dr G. Sangster and Dr J.A. Gray, **95–6**; Dr I. Sarkany, **43**; Professor P. Schever, **425**; Professor C. Scully, **398**; Mr J.C. Smale, **399**; Dr O.D. Standen, **172**; Dr H. Stern, **294–5**, **482**; Dr J. Stevenson, **382–4**; Dr R.N.P. Sutton, **270–1**, **182**, **322**, **324**, **326**,

337–8, 379–80, **401**; Dr Frances Tatnell, **491**; Dr M.M. Esiri and Dr A.H. Tomlinson and the Editor of the *Journal of The Neurological Sciences*, **236**; Dr A.H. Tomlinson, **275–6**; Dr J.M. Vetters and the Department of Pathology, University of Glasgow, **40**, **51**, **101–2**, **134–5**, **169**, **208–9**, **235**, **237**, **274**, **296**, **312–14**, **323**, **339–42**, **445**, **484**, **488**; Dr R.V. Walley, **170**; Dr J.F. Warin, **117–18**; Dr D.A. Warrell, **161**, **400**, **402–3**; Dr D.I. Weiss and the Editor, *American Journal of Diseases of Childhood*, **375**; Dr P. Welsby, **396–7**; Department of Pathology, Whittington Hospital, **69**; Dr P.H.A. Willcox, **416–17**; Dr I. Zamiri, **127**, **129**.

We wish to express special thanks to our colleagues, Dr A.M. Ramsay and Dr Hillas Smith, in the Infectious Diseases Department of The Royal Free Hospital, and to Dr J.I. Pugh of The City Hospital, St Albans, for their help and advice in preparing this atlas. We are also indebted to Dr C.S. Ratnatunga of The Royal Free Hospital and to Mr Martin Jones of the Photographic Department of the North London Group of Hospitals. Many of the colour reproductions have been obtained from members of the Association for the Study of Infectious Disease, to whom we are most grateful. We would also like to thank Dr Susan Young for her assistance in reading and criticising the proofs. Every endeavour has been made to identify the source of the illustrations, but if any mistakes have been made we offer our sincere apologies.

PREFACE

The twentieth century has witnessed tremendous advances in the understanding of infectious disease, but many problems remain. With the natural ebb and flow of infection some old plagues have vanished; while others have been routed by rising standards of living and great advances in preventive medicine. Yet experience teaches that there is no final victory over infection, for elimination of one problem highlights another, and the delicate balance between man and micro-organism remains. Moreover, the speed of air travel is such that banished infections can readily invade from distant lands. Constant vigilance is essential, but few undergraduates have the opportunity to study infectious diseases at the bedside and most enter their profession ill-equipped to recognise even common infections, which form such an important part of everyday practice.

This atlas endeavours to provide the student and newly qualified doctor with a guide to the diagnosis of the common exanthemata, and the experienced physician with clinical photographs of less common though important diseases. It is not feasible to encompass the whole of the subject in one atlas, for many conditions are rare and others do not lend themselves to photographic illustration. Emphasis has been placed on the clinical aspects of disease, but this would be incomplete without a brief account of the causative organism and the relevant pathology. The texts accompanying the illustrations are of necessity short, but, when read in sequence, are intended to give a simple, coherent account of each disease. When size is important in an illustration the relevant information is provided in the text.

MILES

Pharmaceutical Division

Miles Inc.
400 Morgan Lane
West Haven, CT 06516
203 937-2000

Dear Doctor:

Miles Inc. Pharmaceutical Division is pleased to be able to provide you with this beautifully illustrated series, <u>The Miles Color Atlas of Infectious Diseases</u>. Distribution of educational material on infectious disease is representative of Miles' ongoing commitment to the practice of medicine. We hope this atlas will be helpful in assisting with your patient communication.

Sincerely,

H. Brian Allen, MD
Director, Scientific Relations

CONTENTS

132 Anginose variety of infectious mononucleosis. The anginose form of infectious mononucleosis is of similar appearance to diphtheria, but the exudate usually retains a striking white hue and does not spread further than the tonsils. Despite the alarming exudate on the tonsils, the patient's general condition remains good. Generalised enlargement of lymph nodes and splenomegaly indicate the correct clinical diagnosis, which is confirmed by finding characteristic mononuclear cells in the blood and a positive Paul–Bunnell test or one of its simplified variants.

133 Laryngeal diphtheria. Diphtheria of the larynx may be primary or secondary to pharyngeal diphtheria. Toxic absorption is slight, and the illness is dominated by respiratory obstruction caused by the membrane. As breathing becomes more difficult the accessory muscles are brought into play, and the soft parts of the chest wall and supraclavicular fossae are sucked inwards. The child becomes restless and frightened as he struggles for breath. Eventually the violent muscular effort can no longer be sustained, the child falls back exhausted, and death swiftly follows.

Diagnosis of laryngeal diphtheria is easy when membrane is visible in the pharynx but otherwise presents difficulty. Viral forms of laryngitis are associated with catarrhal signs in other parts of the respiratory tract and generally have a more abrupt onset than diphtheria.

134 Histological changes in diphtheritic tracheobronchitis. Diphtheria bacilli, multiplying on the respiratory mucosa, provoke an inflammatory response. The superficial tissues become infiltrated by leucocytes and fibrin-rich fluid exudes from the engorged vessels. The epithelial cells die and are enmeshed with the bacteria in a coagulum of protein to form a membrane. In the lower respiratory tract, where the ciliated epithelium is loosely attached, the membrane is easily dislodged and may be coughed out at tracheotomy or impacted in the larynx. (A = membrane, B = submucosa infiltrated by leucocytes, C = cartilage ring.)

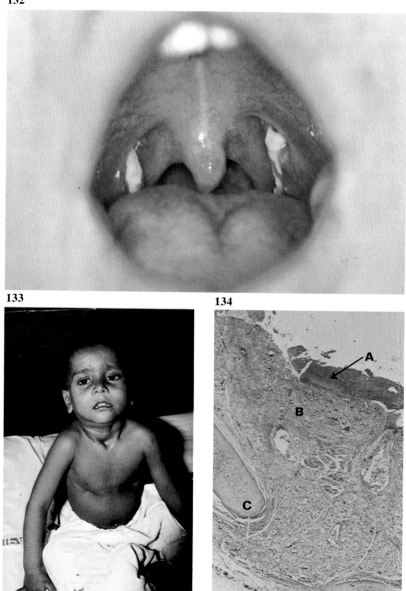

135 Histology of the heart in diphtheria. Diphtheria toxin appears to act primarily on cardiac muscle cells causing fatty degeneration. These patchy areas of damaged myocardium soon become surrounded and infiltrated by leucocytes, many of which are macrophages. In surviving patients fibroblastic repair results in microscopical scars but these do not seem to impair cardiac function.

136 Electrocardiographic changes in diphtheria. Toxic damage to the heart manifests clinically about the eighth to tenth day but may appear earlier in severe cases. The first signs are tachycardia and an irregular pulse. Inversion of T waves or alterations in the ST segment are to be expected in the early stage, and complete heart block may ensue. Restlessness, pallor, vomiting, precordial pain and oliguria are grave prognostic signs. Death commonly occurs about the fifteenth day; survival beyond this stage makes the outlook more hopeful.

This electrocardiogram shows severe changes in a fatal case of diphtheria caused by a mitis stain. Nodal bradycardia is present with ventricular ectopic escape, depression of the ST segment, and inversion of T waves.

135

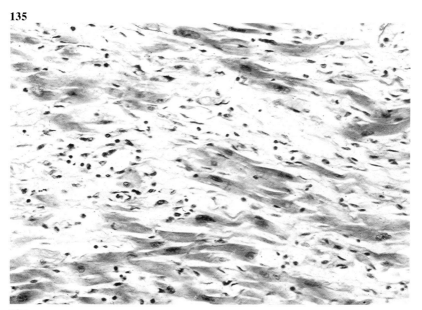

136

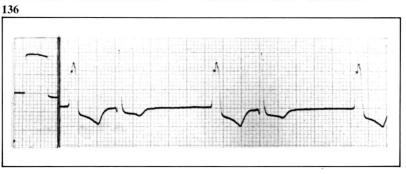

Vincent's infection

137 Vincent's organisms. Dilute carbol fuchsin. A spirochaete and fusiform bacillus are found in large numbers in certain mouth lesions and in ulcerative or necrotic lesions elsewhere. The spirochaete, *Borrelia vincentii*, measures 7 to 18μm in length and has three to eight loose, open coils. It is actively motile and is an obligate anaerobe. The associated bacillus, *Fusobacterium fusiforme*, is cigar-shaped and measures 5 to 14μm. It is non-motile and a strict anaerobe. Both organisms are easily detected in smears, stained by dilute carbol fuchsin, but are difficult to culture.

138 Vincent's angina. Vincent's organisms may be found in small numbers on healthy gums. They do not usually act as primary pathogens but as secondary invaders when superficial tissues have been damaged or are defective as a result of trauma, other infections, malnutrition, agranulocytosis or leukaemia. In temperate climates infection is confined to the buccal cavity or respiratory tract, but in tropical climates the organisms may be found in skin ulcers (see **356**).

In Vincent's angina membranous ulcers may be present on the tonsils or pharynx. Halitosis is a feature, but general disturbance is slight. Infection may spread to adjacent areas of the palate.

139 Acute ulcerative gingivitis. When the gums are involved there is destruction of the interdental papillae, leaving shallow concave ulcers with white necrotic margins. Vincent's infection may cause widespread destruction with extensive ulceration. The regional lymph nodes are enlarged.

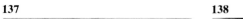

137

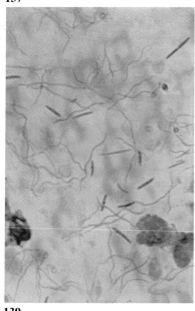

138

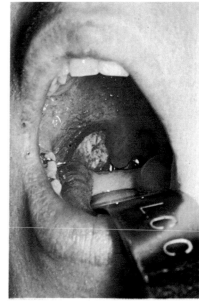

139

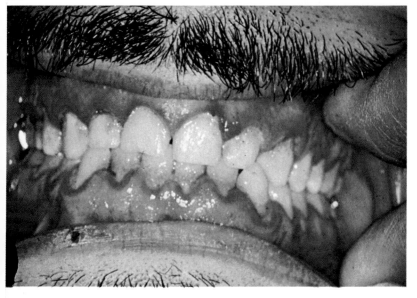

Thrush

140 *Candida albicans*. When conditions are favourable the fungus appears as spherical or oval yeast cells, called blastospores, which reproduce by budding. When conditions are less favourable it grows as a pseudomycelium of non-branching, filamentous cells, which divide by constriction. Further yeast cells are formed by budding at these division sites; both forms are thin-walled. Some yeast cells become larger, develop thick walls, and enter a resting phase. These resting cells are termed chlamydospores. *C. albicans* is Gram positive.

141 *Candida albicans*. **Gram stain of smear from 48 hour growth on blood agar at 37°C.** *Candida albicans* is a yeast-like fungus found in man, animals and birds. It is a common surface commensal in man and is present in the mouth and faeces of 20 to 30% of healthy people. Superficial infection of skin or mucous membranes occurs in debilitated patients or when there has been local disturbance as a result of infection or antibiotic treatment. Deep-seated infections and chronic superficial infections may complicate disorders of immunity.

142 **Oral thrush.** Thrush infection of the mouth may occur in infants as a result of cross-infection from the mother or from other infants, especially in bottle-fed babies. In adults, infection is usually endogenous and is found in dehydrated or debilitated patients, or when the bacterial flora of the buccal cavity has been disturbed by antibiotic therapy. The raw inflamed mucous membrane is covered with patches of creamy-white exudate.

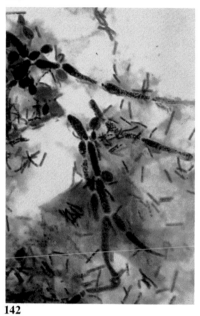

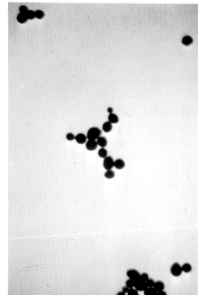

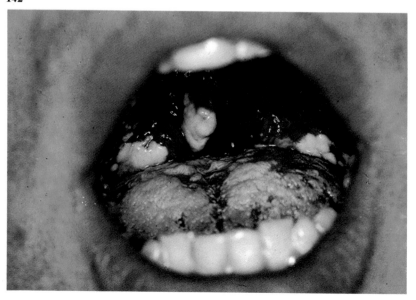

143 Chronic oral thrush. Chronic infection of the mouth may be associated with immunodeficiency, such as the acquired immune deficiency syndrome (AIDS). Firm, diffuse, white plaques or numerous white papules with intervening erythema may be found in the buccal cavity and persist for months or even years depending on the nature of the underlying deficiency.

144 Vulvovaginitis. Nappy rash in babies may be caused by candida and is particularly common in those with diarrhoea or those receiving antibiotic treatment. The rash starts round the anus and spreads over the perineum affecting skin in contact with the nappy. There is a well-defined area of redness with raised edges. Satellite lesions may begin as small pustules that rupture to leave small raw patches. The skin is macerated. In an ammoniacal rash the skin folds tend to be spared.

Genital thrush may prove troublesome in women using oral contraceptives or during pregnancy. Redness of the vagina and labia may be accompanied by severe pruritus and scanty or thick white discharge.

143

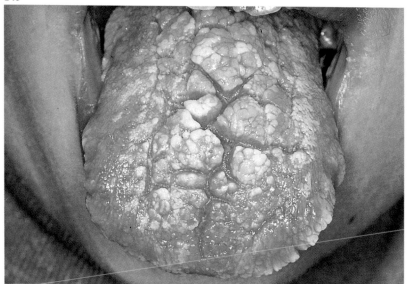

144

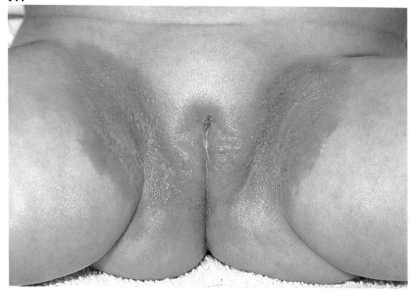

145 Balanitis. Poor hygiene may result in severe irritation of the foreskin and glans with blistering and patches of thrush.

146 Paronychia. Candida infection may spread from the nail fold under the adjacent nail causing deformity and even loss of the nail. It is especially common in those whose hands are frequently immersed in water, and in patients with diabetes or endocrine disorders. Nail infection as a manifestation of chronic mucocutaneous candidiasis may occur in patients with immunological defects. In this child the infection was caused by persistent thumb-sucking.

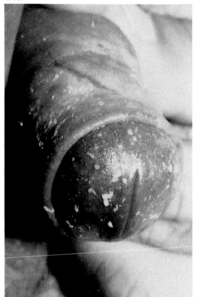

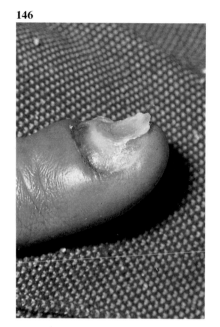

Leprosy

Leprosy is caused by *Mycobacterium leprae*, and man is the only natural host. The disease is found mainly in the tropics and subtropics. Close and continuous household contact is necessary for spread, and infection is usually derived from the nasal discharges of an infectious patient. Most infected people do not develop the disease; in those who do, the pattern of disease exhibits a spectrum from the tuberculoid, showing notable delayed hypersensitivity, to the lepromatous, in which there is virtually no cellular reaction by the host.

147 Organism — *M. leprae*. This is a slender acid-fast bacillus, which has not been cultured on media or in tissue culture, but grows exceedingly slowly in the footpads of mice and armadillos. It replicates with a doubling time of about 13 days, and is an obligate intracellular parasite found in macrophages. The large number of organisms in this section of skin suggests that the patient had lepromatous leprosy.

148 Histology. The Schwann cells of peripheral nerves, being phagocytic, may contain bacteria. When there is a host response a granuloma is formed, consisting of epithelioid cells and giant cells surrounded by lymphocytes. As a result, the nerve may be compressed and damaged. Depending on the individual nerve this may result in motor or sensory disturbance or both.

149 Lepromin reaction at four weeks. The lepromin reaction is a skin reaction observed after the intradermal injection of an extract of leprosy bacilli. It is of delayed hypersensitivity type but differs from the tuberculin reaction in that it is seen after several weeks rather than 48 hours. It is strongly positive in patients with tuberculoid leprosy and negative in those towards and at the lepromatous end of the spectrum.

147

148 **149**

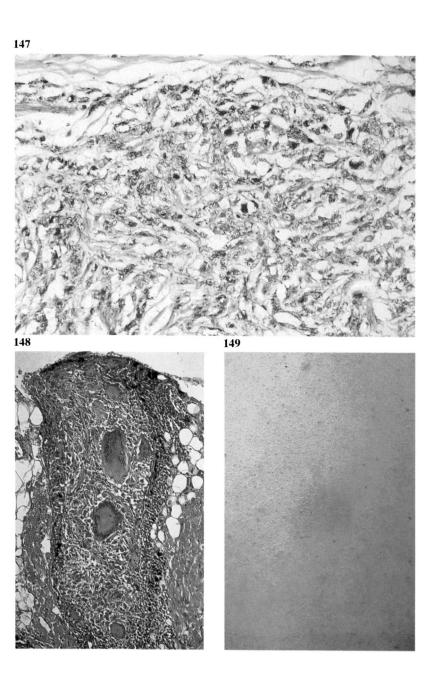

150 Appearance of face. The leonine facies is characteristic of lepromatous leprosy. The skin is thickened and ridged, the nose widened, and the ear lobes also thickened. Bacilli are readily found in large numbers in skin smears and also in the nodules shown here.

151 Erythema nodosum leprosum (ENL). Patients with lepromatous leprosy often suffer from ENL. The eruption is painful and consists of multiple reddened cutaneous nodules. It may be accompanied by constitutional upset, proteinuria, and orchitis. The incidence and severity of attacks vary greatly between patients, and may be precipitated by a variety of circumstances, including emotional factors. The underlying pathology is thought to be a vasculitis secondary to immune complex deposition.

152 'Upgrading' reaction. Patients whose disease is not at the two extremes of the spectrum may move their position in the spectrum according to their response to the organisms. Here, a patient towards the lepromatous end is showing more response than previously and is moving away from the lepromatous end in an upgrading reaction. Clinically, this is seen as areas of erythema. Although this reaction may be considered as protective in nature, the increased cellular response may result in nerve compression and an increase in neurological findings.

150

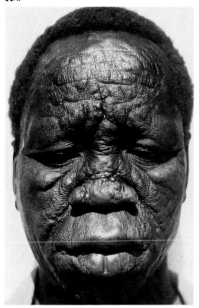

151

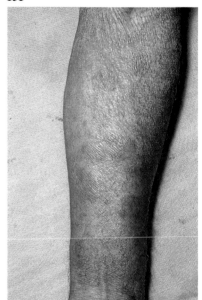

152

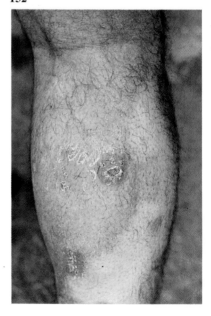

153 Tuberculoid leprosy. This patient is categorised towards the tuberculoid end of the immunological spectrum. Skin lesions are relatively few, asymmetrical, raised, anaesthetic, and do not sweat. Organisms are very scanty. Histologically the lesion is a granuloma; the lepromin test is strongly positive.

154 Nerve infection. In some patients the disease is purely neural and no skin lesions are seen. In this patient the radial nerve is affected causing wrist drop and anaesthesia of the thumb.

153

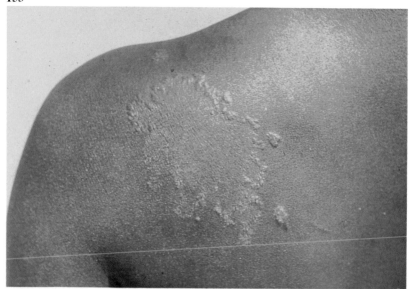

154

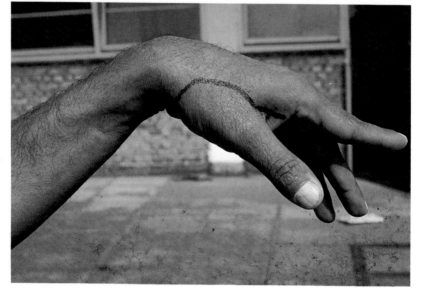

155   Claw hand. Claw hand is a characteristic feature of leprosy, especially in those patients categorised in the middle of the spectrum with borderline disease. The ulnar nerve is affected; patients are unable to flex the metacarpophalangeal joints, and there is prominent wasting of the thenar and hypothenar eminences. The deformity may be aggravated by subsequent contractures. Sensory loss is present in the ulnar distribution.

156   Ulcers. Ulcers of the feet are common in leprosy. They may be perforating ulcers of the sole, similar to those seen in diabetes, or round the ankle, as seen here. Because of anaesthesia the foot is vulnerable to damage from prolonged pressure, burns, or general injuries. The ulcers are slow to heal and tend to break down; they may be associated with considerable loss of tissue, scarring, and deformity.

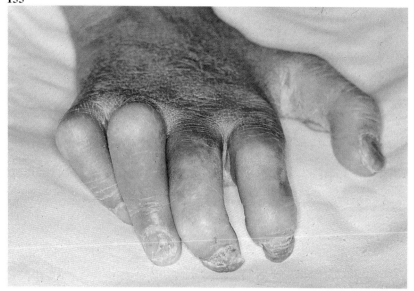

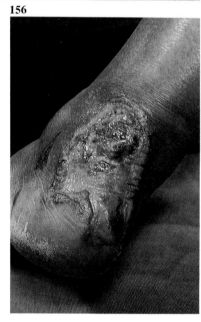

Tetanus

157 *Clostridium tetani* (**negative stain with nigrosin**). The tetanus organism is ubiquitous, being present in soil and dust, though the degree of contamination varies from district to district. It is often found in the intestinal tract of animals and sometimes in man. *Clostridium tetani* is a Gram-positive rod measuring $2.5\,\mu$m in length and is a strict anaerobe. It forms spherical terminal spores, highly resistant to heat and disinfectants.

The vegetative bacillus produces a powerful exotoxin with a special affinity for nervous tissue. The organism usually gains access through a wound and multiplies locally in the damaged tissues, producing exotoxin. This is absorbed and conveyed to the nervous system, where it disturbs the regulation of reflex arcs and abolishes reciprocal innervation. Consequently afferent stimuli produce an exaggerated response.

158 **Trismus.** The first evidence of tetanus is usually difficulty in opening the mouth because of increased tone in the masseters. At this early stage mumps may be suspected, but hypertonus can generally be detected elsewhere, and there is no evidence of salivary gland involvement.

Pain and stiffness in the neck and back may simulate meningitis, but the correct diagnosis soon becomes apparent as the disease advances.

157

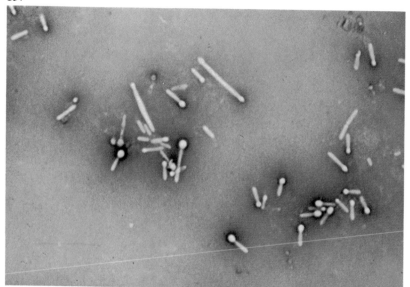

158

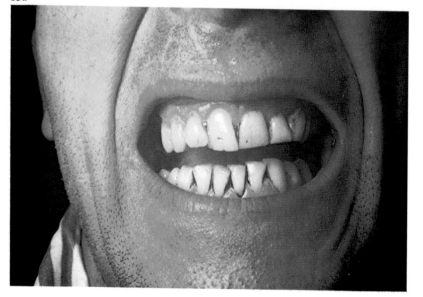

133

159 Risus sardonicus. Spasm of the facial muscles causes retraction of the angles of mouth to expose the clenched teeth in a characteristic snarling grin.

160 Opisthotonus in a child. Tetanus toxin causes overactivity of motor nerve cells resulting in muscle rigidity and spasm. Tonic rigidity is present in every case and persists throughout the illness. When the spinal muscles are severely affected opisthotonus results. In mild attacks the disease may be arrested at the stage of rigidity, and spasms do not develop.

If the disease advances spasms appear and become progressively more frequent and severe. With the onset of a convulsion the whole body is suddenly thrown into a violent spasm by the sustained contraction of all somatic muscles. The jaws are tightly clenched, the back arched, and the limbs are usually extended. Each paroxysm may be accompanied by muscle cramp so severe that the patient lies in dread of the next attack. Patients remain fully conscious throughout their terrifying ordeal.

161 Tetanus neonatorum. The stump of the umbilical cord may be infected by the use of non-sterile instruments or dressings and this may lead to neonatal tetanus. Failure to suck is an early sign and this is followed by hypertonus and muscle spasms. Despite treatment mortality is often greater than 50%.

159

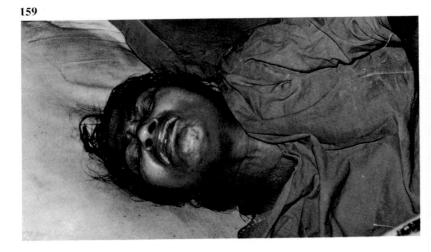

160

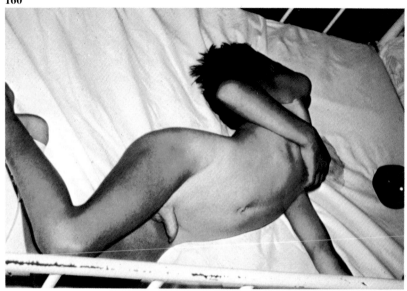

161

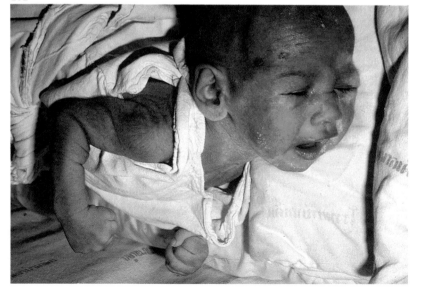

Anthrax

162 Smear from culture of anthrax bacilli. Anthrax is primarily a disease of animals, caused by a bacillus that forms highly resistant spores on exposure to oxygen. In tropical countries, where climatic conditions favour rapid sporulation with heavy contamination of soil, anthrax is mainly spread from infected pasture. In temperate zones sporulation is less rapid, and vegetative bacilli are readily destroyed by soil bacteria; therefore contamination is slight. Under these conditions anthrax is seldom acquired from grazing and is usually derived from imported foodstuffs. Sheep, cattle, horses and goats are very susceptible.

The anthrax bacillus is a non-motile, Gram-positive rod. It measures 4 to $10\,\mu$m in length by 1 to $1\cdot5\,\mu$m in width and is one of the largest of the pathogenic bacteria. In smears from infected animals the bacilli are encapsulated and lie singly or in short chains, but in cultures on nutrient agar capsules are not formed and the organism is arranged in long strands. When exposed to oxygen it forms spores that are oval in shape with a double-layered outer membrane.

163 Anthrax bacilli in pulmonary capillaries. Gram stain (x 880). Pulmonary anthrax or wool-sorter's disease is a rare condition in man, acquired by inhaling anthrax spores in dust from infected wool or hair. The onset is abrupt and the illness follows a swift course with frequent haemoptyses and acute respiratory distress culminating in death within two or three days.

On postmortem examination there is severe pulmonary oedema with widespread haemorrhagic bronchopneumonia. Large numbers of anthrax bacilli are present and are very conspicuous in Gram-stained preparations because of their large size and deep blue colour.

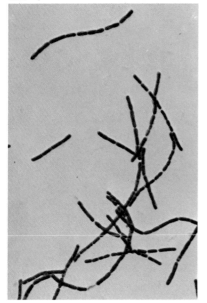

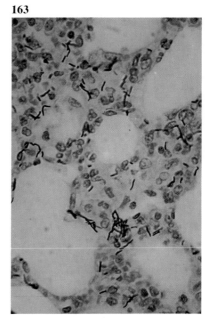

164   Cutaneous anthrax (malignant pustule). Early lesion on neck. The skin is involved in 98% of human infections, and lesions are found most commonly on exposed areas of the body. Cutaneous anthrax is chiefly an occupational disease. Infection may be acquired directly from animals, but it is derived more commonly from hides, wool, hair, raw bonemeal or other animal products.

Anthrax of the neck is an occupational disease of hide porters. An itchy papule develops at the site of entry and is surrounded within a day or two by a ring of haemorrhagic vesicles. Oedema is a striking feature in cutaneous anthrax. It commences round the original lesion and spreads extensively wherever the subcutaneous tissues are lax. The skin may retain its normal colour or become intensely red. Blood cultures may prove positive.

165   Anthrax lesion on neck. As the lesion progresses the central area ulcerates and dries, forming a thick, leathery, dark scab which later extends into the vesicular zone. The crust is firmly attached to the underlying tissues and gradually separates over a period of two or three weeks, leaving a deep ulcer which slowly fills with granulation tissue. The lesion is painless and pus seldom forms, except on rare occasions when there is secondary infection. Before the introduction of antibiotic treatment mortality from anthrax of the neck was much greater than from anthrax of the forehead.

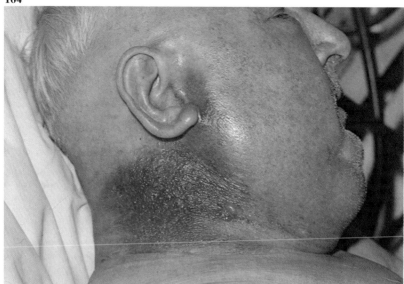

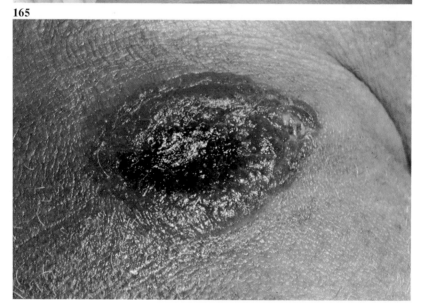

166   Anthrax of forearm. This may occur in butchers handling infected carcases or in gardeners using contaminated bonemeal. Oedema may be slight. This illustration shows the eschar beginning to separate.

167   Anthrax of back. The lower limb and trunk are affected in only 1·9% of cases. The patient opposite worked in a factory manufacturing paint brushes. She developed a large lesion over her left scapula, but there was very little constitutional disturbance. By the time the photograph was taken the vesicles had already ruptured and had been incorporated in the eschar, which was firmly adherent.

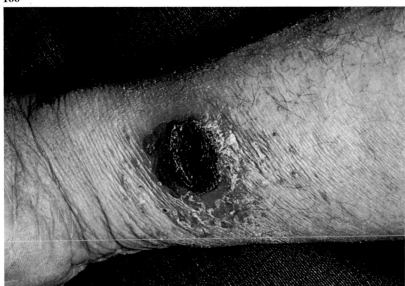

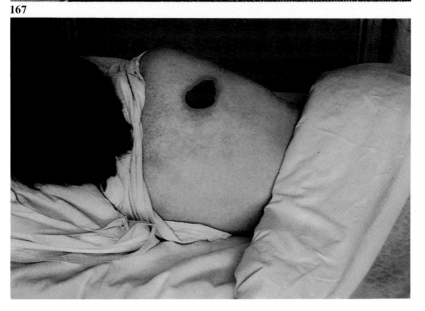

Leptospirosis

168 Smear from culture of *Leptospira icterohaemorrhagiae* (silver impregnation stain). The genus *Leptospira* includes two main species: *L. interrogens* and *L. biflexa*. Both species contain many serotypes (serovars), some of which are pathogenic, and others saprophytic. Parasitic leptospires are indistinguishable from one another morphologically or culturally but can be classified serologically. More than 50 serotypes have already been identified. Leptospires are about 7 to 14 μm long and have a closely coiled body with hooked ends. On electron microscopy the cytoplasm is seen to be wound round a single, straight and stiff axostyle. The organism is actively motile. It is an aerobe, and parasitic strains grow readily on fluid culture medium containing animal serum.

Leptospirosis is a zoonosis affecting rodents, dogs, cats, pigs and cattle. Leptospires may cause little harm to the primary host, where they colonise the renal tubules and are shed in large numbers in the urine. Man and susceptible animals may be infected indirectly by water or articles contaminated by such urine. The organism enters through minor breaches in the skin or mucosa. Farm workers and sewage workers are at special risk.

169 Section of liver showing leptospires (silver impregnation). There is no obvious reaction at the portal of entry, and the organisms quickly enter the bloodstream. When death occurs during the first week of illness leptospires can be found in many tissues but subsequently they are most easily detected in the kidneys. They are best demonstrated by fluorescent antibody technique.

There is a striking contrast between the depth of jaundice in severe cases of leptospirosis and the histological changes in the liver. Damage to the liver cells is much less severe than in viral hepatitis, and the serum transaminase activity is often only slightly increased. Cholestasis is the most prominent feature. In postmortem preparations the parenchymal cells are seen to be separated from each other, and there is a high incidence of mitotic figures.

In this section, stained by Levaditi's silver impregnation method, a large number of leptospires with characteristic closely wound spirals can be seen scattered between the liver cells. (Arrow = leptospire.)

168

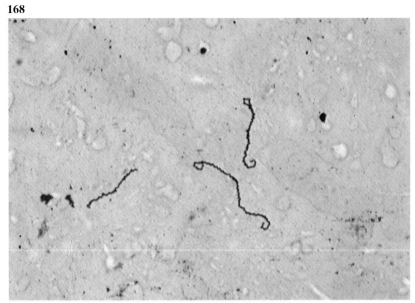

169

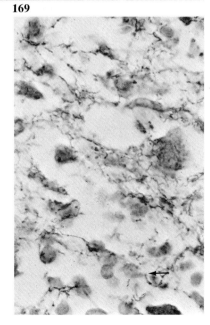

170 **Suffusion of conjunctivae.** Leptospirosis in man is associated with a wide range of clinical syndromes, including classical Weil's disease, aseptic meningitis, influenza-like illness, and unexplained fever. The onset is abrupt with shivering followed by fever. Headache, myalgia and arthralgia are common features. Conjunctival suffusion is often present and may be accompanied by photophobia. Prostration tends to be severe and disproportionate to the physical signs.

171 **Close-up of eye in canicola fever.** Human beings usually develop canicola fever through contact with pig or dog urine containing *L. canicola*, although the leptospire is sometimes found in other animals. Severe and intractable headache is an outstanding and distressing symptom. An aseptic form of meningitis is present in 75% of patients. Roughly 20% have jaundice or evidence of renal damage. Nearly 50% have injection of the conjunctivae.

170

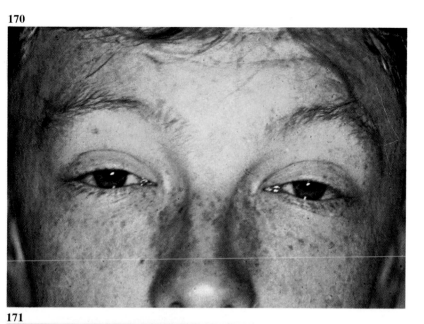

171

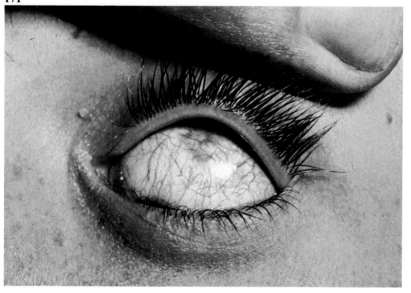

172 Severe Weil's disease. Weil's disease is a severe form of leptospirosis with both hepatic and renal damage. It is commonly caused by *L. icterohaemorrhagiae* derived from rats, but other serotypes have been incriminated. The syndrome is comparatively rare, occurring in roughly 15% of leptospiral infections in man. Even with this most virulent serotype, mild or inapparent infections are not uncommon.

The first week of illness is dominated by fever, headache, severe debility, and muscular pains. Nausea and vomiting may be accompanied by haematemesis, and abdominal pain may be so severe that a surgical emergency is suspected. Jaundice may be the earliest sign but may not develop until the end of the first week. At the same time haemorrhages may appear in the skin and mucous membranes and, if profuse, indicate an unfavourable prognosis. The second week is critical. Jaundice deepens, haemorrhages increase, and renal failure develops. Most deaths take place at this stage from renal failure and some lives may be saved by effective dialysis. During the third week the illness abates, renal function improves, and jaundice lessens. Eventually full renal and hepatic function is restored.

173 Face in Weil's disease. Haemorrhages are common in severely ill patients with jaundice and renal failure. Petechiae or ecchymoses may be found in skin, conjunctivae, or mucous membranes. Epistaxis may be a presenting feature, and there may be profuse bleeding into the bowel during the second week. Mild haemoptysis is not unusual.

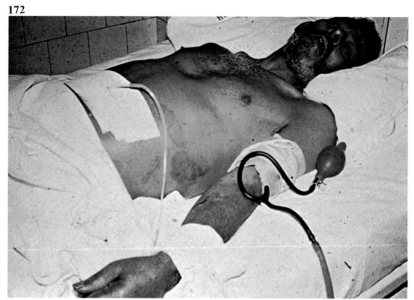

172

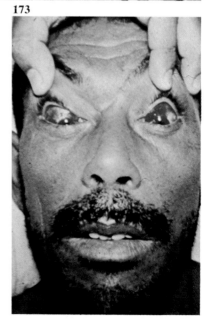

173

Gonorrhoea

Gonorrhoea is caused by *Neisseria gonorrhoeae*, an infection confined to humans. In adults it is transmitted by sexual contact; in children by non-sexual contact or by fomites. Gonorrhoea in adults may manifest as local infection of the urogenital tract, rectum, conjunctiva or oropharynx, or generalised infection of the skin, joints, meninges, and endocardium. Transmission from the mother during delivery may result in acute conjunctivitis; contamination of flannels and towels may cause acute vulvovaginitis in young girls.

174 Smear of organism (Gram stain). *Neisseria gonorrhoeae* is a Gram-negative bacterium, usually sensitive to human serum and readily ingested by neutrophil polymorphonuclear leucocytes, as seen in this smear stained with Gram stain, where they appear as intracellular diplococci. They have fastidious growth requirements.

175 Urethritis. This is the commonest presentation of gonorrhoea in men. A purulent urethral discharge appears within a few days after exposure and is associated with dysuria. Untreated, this will often last for many weeks before clearing spontaneously. The persistent inflammation predisposes to urethral stricture. Gonococcal urethritis is clinically indistinguishable from non-gonococcal urethritis caused by chlamydia, but can be differentiated by examination of a urethral smear. Painful lymphadenitis is present in 15% of cases. Proctitis may be the presenting feature in homosexuals.

176 Cervicitis. Symptoms are absent in 80% of women infected with the gonococcus. An infected cervix may have a normal appearance with mucoid discharge or may be inflamed with mucopurulent or profuse purulent discharge. The urethra or rectum may be infected from the vaginal discharge. Pelvic spread may result in endometritis, salpingitis, or peritonitis.

177 Bartholin's abscess. A more dramatic presentation in women is infection of Bartholin's gland. The lymphadenitis is usually unilateral and may progress to form abscesses. Skene's glands may also be affected.

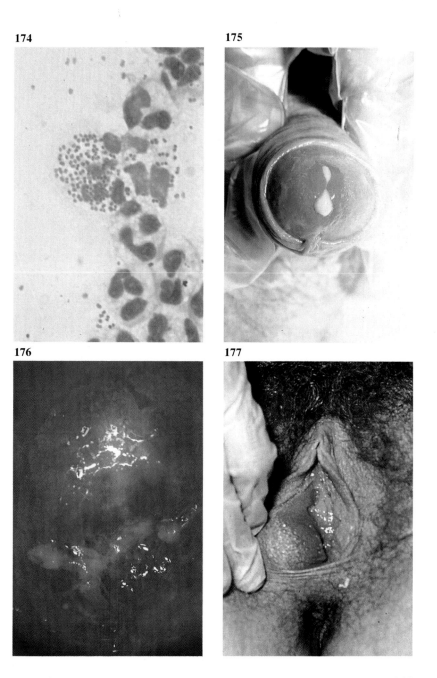

178 Gonorrhoea — skin lesions. Disseminated infection is caused by strains of gonococci resistant to serum and accounts for 2% of all gonococcal infection. It is more common in women. Bacteraemia may lead to septic arthritis, tenosynovitis, meningitis, endocarditis or skin lesions. Skin lesions are the most common feature and consist of a sparse rash over the limbs, sparing the face and trunk.

179 Gonorrhoea — skin lesion. The most characteristic lesion is a pustule on an erythematous base. Slight fever is common. Some patients may have no constitutional upset; others may be very ill with a high fever.

180 Gonorrhoea — skin lesion. The skin lesions vary and may consist of macules, papules, pustules, haemorrhagic bullae, or necrotic lesions as shown here. The organism is seldom grown from the skin lesions but may be cultured from blood or purulent joint effusions. Most patients have migratory arthralgia during the first week mainly affecting the large joints. In some cases, this will progress to septic arthritis. Tenosynovitis is found in about 25% of cases.

181 Conjunctivitis. Ophthalmia may result from direct contact with an infected birth canal. It follows two to five days after birth and may cause septicaemia. Transfer of infection from discharges elsewhere may cause conjunctivitis in adults. Young girls living in overcrowded conditions are very susceptible to gonococcal vulvovaginitis spread by moist articles such as flannels or towels. Infection is very seldom spread by fomites to adults.

178

179

180

181

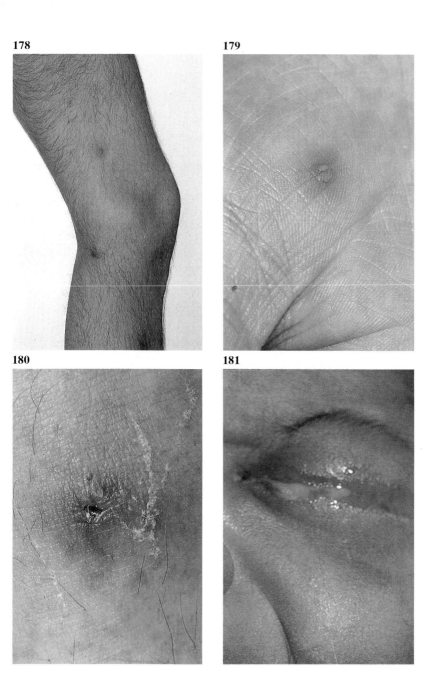

Chlamydial infection

Chlamydia are intracellular parasites, whose genome contains both DNA and RNA. They are considered to be specialised bacteria with a complex form of replication ending in binary fission, and can be divided into two groups sharing a complement-fixing antigen. *Chlamydia trachomatis* (group A) is responsible for genital infections, conjunctivitis at any age and pneumonitis in infancy; *Chlamydia psittaci* (group B) causes ornithosis.

182 Chlamydial infection — conjunctival smear. Conjunctival scrapings from patients with neonatal inclusion conjunctivitis, when stained by Giemsa's method, may show intracytoplasmic basophilic inclusion bodies. The technique is less sensitive in adult inclusion conjunctivitis, and of little or no value in genital infection. Tissue cultures, using pretreated cells, such as McCoy, are more reliable. Humoral antibody may be detected by immunofluorescence, but the results of serological tests must be interpreted with caution.

183 Conjunctivitis in newborn baby. Infection of the eye from the mother's cervix at the time of birth may result in inclusion conjunctivitis of the newborn. A mucopurulent conjunctivitis develops within two weeks of birth and may affect one or both eyes. There are no distinguishing features. The acute stage settles after two weeks or so, but the eye may take several months to return to normal and the disease may progress to mild trachoma.

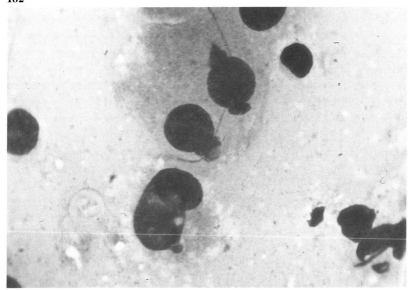

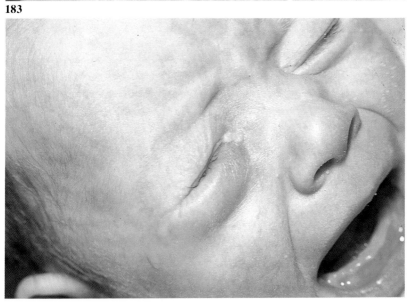

184   Conjunctivitis — adult. Inclusion conjunctivitis in adults also has an acute onset and is accompanied by mucopurulent discharge, conjunctival follicles and superficial punctate keratitis. The follicles are always more prominent in the lower than the upper lid, and appear as rounded swellings, 1 to 2 mm in diameter, which are formed by lymphocytic foci in the subepithelial adenoid layer. Healing takes place slowly over a period of one to two years.

185   Trachoma. Trachoma is also caused by TRIC or non-LGV strains of *Chlamydia trachomatis*. The disease is endemic in many parts of the world where people are crowded together under conditions of poor hygiene. Infection is transmitted by conjunctival secretions, which are transferred on fingers or towels and, above all, by flies. The onset is usually subacute and the course is determined by the presence or absence of secondary infection. The conjunctiva is inflamed and follicles appear in the fornices. They spread over the palpebral conjunctiva but rarely on to the bulbar conjunctiva, and may measure up to 5 mm in diameter. Trachomatous infiltration may extend deeply into the subepithelial tissues of the palpebral conjunctiva. The cornea is affected at an early stage with a superficial keratitis, which is most marked in the upper part. As the disease progresses the conjunctiva becomes scarred and pannus develops, with cloudiness and vascularization of the cornea.

184

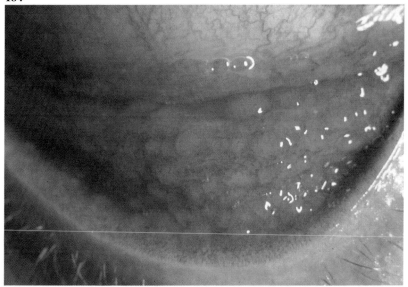

185

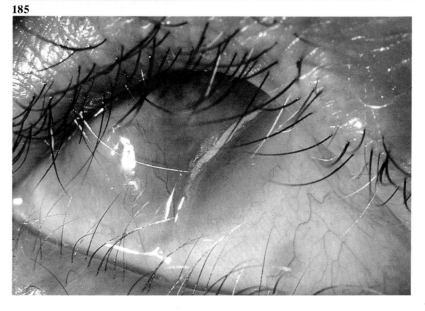

186 Urethritis. *Chlamydia trachomatis* may be isolated from the urethra in up to 5% of symptomless men, 20% of men with gonorrhoea, and 30 to 50% of men with non-specific urethritis. Chlamydial urethritis is clinically indistinguishable from gonococcal, though it tends to be milder. Chlamydial infection is also associated with epididymitis and with Reiter's disease.

187 Cervicitis. Chlamydial infections are common in women: the organism has been detected in up to 5% of healthy women, and up to 60% of women with gonorrhoea. Chlamydial cervicitis is accompanied by mucopurulent discharge from the os and the cervix is reddened and oedematous. Chlamydia is responsible for some cases of salpingitis and proctitis in women. Infection acquired at birth may give rise to inclusion conjunctivitis in the newborn baby, or pneumonitis in the infant.

188 Lymphogranuloma venereum. This sexually transmitted disease is caused by the LGV strain of *Chlamydia trachomatis*. After an incubation period of one to three weeks a primary lesion may be detected on the genitalia in about 10% of patients. This consists of a small papule or vesicle, which may ulcerate, but heals within a few days without leaving a scar.

After two to ten weeks the patient enters the secondary stage, with painful swelling of the regional lymph nodes. This is occasionally accompanied by constitutional disturbance, with fever, headache and arthralgia. As the disease progresses the lymph nodes become matted and attached to the overlying skin, which is reddened. The buboes may suppurate and discharge through sinuses on to the surface of the skin, vagina or bowel.

The disease may resolve after three to four months, or may advance to the third stage, with strictures of the urethra, vagina or rectum. Fistulae or perirectal abscesses may prove troublesome and lymphatic obstruction may result in chronic oedema with enlargement of the penis or vulva.

186

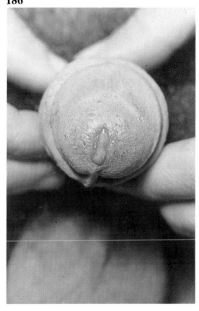

187

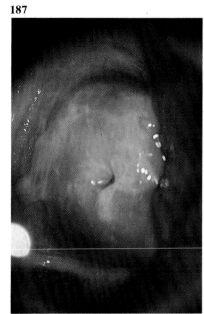

188

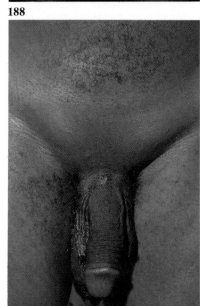

157

189 Ornithosis. This is a worldwide zoonosis caused by *Chlamydia psittaci*. Infection is common in humans occupationally exposed to psittacine birds in pet shops and aviaries, and other birds in turkey- and duck-processing plants. Infection is rarely transmitted from humans.

Much infection is subclinical or mild, resembling influenza. Severe attacks begin with an influenza-like illness. During the first week the patient has a high fever with relative bradycardia and possible gastro-intestinal disturbance with diarrhoea. A dry cough may be present, but there are few chest signs. Evidence of consolidation may appear during the second week, and the extent of the pneumonia or radiological examination is disproportionate to the physical signs. The radiographic appearances are not diagnostic. The erythrocyte sedimentation rate tends to be notably increased, and the diagnosis is confirmed by serological tests. The illness subsides after 7 to 14 days, but convalescence tends to be protracted, and radiological clearance may take several weeks.

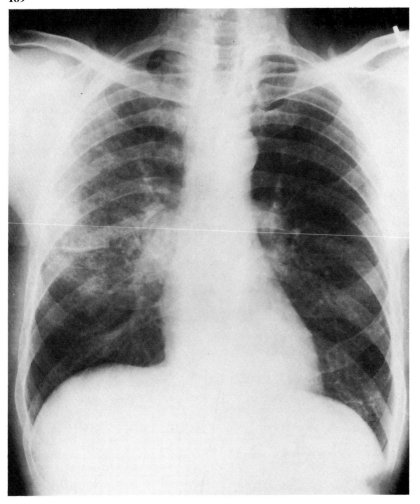

Syphilis

Syphilis is caused by the spirochaete *Treponema pallidum*. Acquired infection is almost entirely transmitted by sexual contact; congenital infection often comes from a mother who has been infected during or shortly before pregnancy. The incidence of syphilis has greatly declined since the introduction of antibiotics.

190   Organism — *Treponema pallidum*. *Treponema pallidum* is a slender spirochaete about $10\,\mu$m in length with roughly 10 turns to its spiral. It has an undulating movement and rotates about its long axis. It is sensitive to drying and dies rapidly above 42°C but can survive for some days at 4°C. It cannot be seen by ordinary microscopy but is best seen by dark-field illumination as shown here; it can be stained by silver in tissue sections. It is a human parasite and is indistinguishable morphologically or serologically from treponemes causing yaws, pinta or bejel.

191   Syphilis — chancre in a male. In heterosexual men the primary lesion of syphilis, the chancre, is most commonly found on the glans penis or in the sulcus and less commonly on the penile shaft. The chancre is indurated but is not tender and is often associated with enlarged but painless inguinal lymph nodes. Dark-field preparations are made from serum exuded from the chancre.

192   Syphilis — chancre in a female. Classically, the chancre appears after an incubation period of 21 to 35 days (extremes 9 to 90 days) as a single lesion in 50% of cases. It evolves rapidly from a macule to a papule, which erodes and forms a round, painless ulcer with a clean surface and surrounding hard induration. It heals within three to ten weeks leaving a thin atrophic scar in some cases. Vulval lesions may be readily recognised, but cervical lesions are commonly overlooked.

193   Syphilis — anal chancre. In homosexual men the anus is a major site for the primary lesion. Anal lesions may also be found in women, and mouth lesions occur in both sexes.

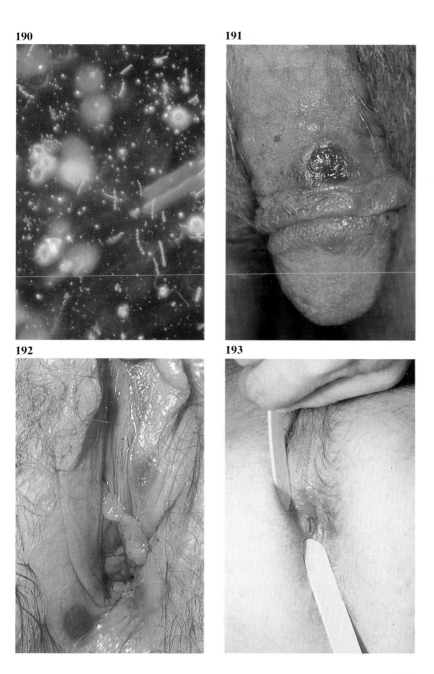

194 Syphilis — rash. A rash is the presenting feature in 70% of cases and usually appears six to eight weeks after infection, when the primary lesion is declining or has healed. It may be accompanied by general symptoms of fever, headache, malaise and arthralgia, and associated with mucous patches, lymphadenitis and meningitis. The rash varies greatly in intensity and appearance. It usually appears first on the trunk and proximal parts of the limbs as discrete pinkish macules, which may evolve into red papules. The lesions do not itch and persist for four to eight weeks.

195 Syphilis — rash. Sometimes the rash may consist of fewer, larger, darker red papules.

196 Syphilis — rash. In a few patients the rash may finally become pustular and form crusts. Lesions of different type may be found on the same patient. Vesicular rashes are not a feature of secondary syphilis.

197 Syphilis — rash. The rash may extend to cover the whole body, including the palms and soles. This distribution should suggest possible secondary syphilis. Involvement of hair follicles may result in patchy alopecia.

When the secondary stage subsides the patient enters the stage of latent syphilis. There is no clinical evidence of active disease, but serological tests remain positive. Some patients with latent syphilis advance to the tertiary stage after an interval of three to ten years or longer.

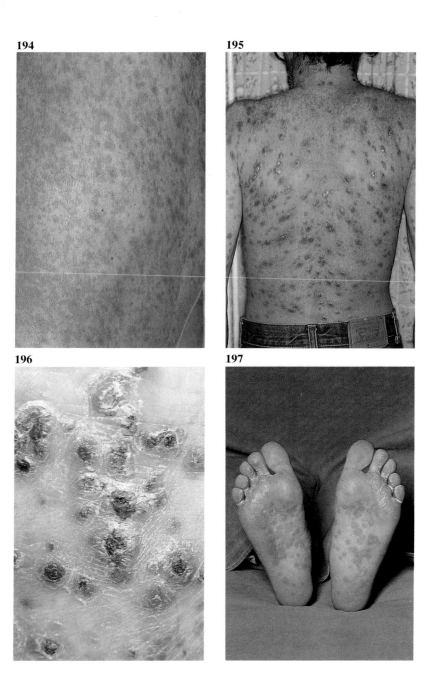

198   Syphilis — chest x-ray showing aneurysm. Before the introduction of penicillin for the treatment of syphilis, between 10 and 40% of patients progressed to the tertiary stage. Cardiovascular disease appeared 10 to 30 years after infection and was accompanied by neuro-syphilis in about 30% of cases. Vasculitis affecting the vasa vasorum of the aorta results in the loss of elastic tissue and subsequent dilatation of the artery. If the root of the aorta is affected the aortic ring becomes dilated causing aortic incompetence.

199   Syphilis — gumma. The basic lesion of tertiary syphilis is a chronic granuloma, known as a gumma. It tends to be localised, asymmetrical in distribution, and destructive in character. A gumma may affect any part of the body. Sometimes a solitary gumma may appear in the sub-cutaneous tissues, increasing in size before breaking down to form a gummatous ulcer. Such an ulcer is painless and has a characteristic appearance. It is roughly circular, with sharply defined 'punched out' edges and an indurated base. A slough of necrotic tissue, like a piece of wash-leather, initially occupies the crater and is firmly adherent. Later, it separates leaving pale granulations. Spirochaetes cannot be detected in the lesion.

200   Congenital syphilis — early manifestations. Congenital syphilis is now extremely rare in developed countries. The clinical course is very variable and in many cases there may be no obvious clinical signs. One of the earliest features may be a mucopurulent nasal discharge, which may persist for many months and is known as the 'snuffles'. Skin eruptions are common during the first two years of life, and there may be evidence of damage to many structures, including mucous mem-branes, bones and teeth.

The rash is most commonly maculopapular and may be followed by extensive sloughing of the epithelium on the palms and soles, and around the mouth and anus. Pemphigoid lesions may be found in congenital syphilis but seldom in acquired syphilis. The skin lesions are teeming with treponema.

These early lesions heal and are followed by a latent period before the late features appear. These include damage to teeth, bones, eyes and auditory nerve as well as gummata and neurosyphilis.

198

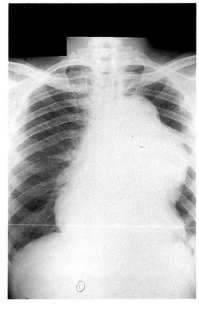

199

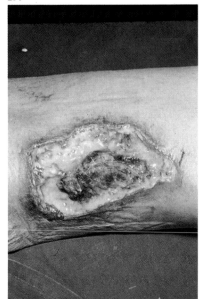

200

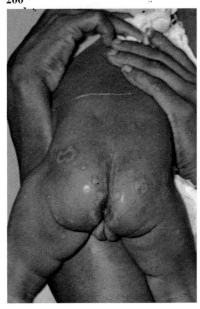

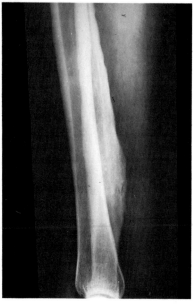

201 Radiograph of tibia and fibula in late form of syphilitic periostitis.
Widespread bone disease is very common in young children with
congenital syphilis and may present as osteochondritis, periostitis, or
osteitis and osteomyelitis, particularly affecting the long bones and the
skull. This early disease may be detected at any time from birth to the
age of three to four years and usually resolves spontaneously.

Bone disease may reappear between the ages of five to 15 years. This
late form is usually very resistant to treatment and may persist indefinitely.
The radiological appearances in syphilitic, tuberculous and chronic
pyogenic bone disease are very similar, and other factors must be taken
into consideration when making a diagnosis. In the juvenile form of
syphilitic periostitis or osteitis new bone may be deposited in lamellated
layers parallel to the shaft or else on the convexity of the shaft. The tibia
is commonly affected, and thickening of the anterior aspect of the
proximal half of the bone may produce the appearance of sabre shin or
tibia.

Chancroid

Chancroid is a sexually transmitted disease caused by the Gram-negative coccobacillus *Haemophilus ducreyi*. As with a number of sexually transmitted diseases, it is more commonly recognised in men than women. The infection is worldwide in distribution and is especially common where social, economic, and hygienic conditions are poor.

Lesions are usually confined to the genitalia and perianal region, with secondary lesions in the inguinal lymph nodes. The initial lesion is a tender papule, which becomes pustular and then erodes to form a non-indurated and painful ulcer. This may coalesce with other lesions, and secondary infection may result in further destruction.

202   Genital lesions in chancroid. Here the penile lesions are associated with greatly enlarged inguinal glands. The lymphadenitis is usually unilateral. The swelling is painful and may rupture to leave a discharging sinus. The penile lesions may be difficult to distinguish from those of granuloma inguinale (Donovanosis). They may also be confused with the primary lesion of syphilis, but can be differentiated by the presence of pain and absence of induration. The two infections coexist in up to 10% of patients, so the possibility of syphilis should always be considered. The diagnosis of chancroid may be confirmed by finding the organism in smears or by culture.

202

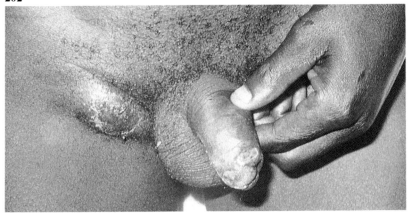

Donovanosis

Donovanosis, granuloma inguinale, and granuloma venereum are names given to the disease produced by *Calymmatobacterium granulomatis,* a Gram-negative encapsulated bacterium, whose relation to other organisms is uncertain. Infection is usually transmitted by sexual contact, but this is not exclusive, as young children may be affected. It is more common in tropical parts of the world.

203 Donovanosis — organism. This is characteristically found in large mononuclear cells and can be demonstrated as deeply staining Donovan bodies in smudge smears made from the lesions. In this smear the preparation was made from the penile lesion. The organism is difficult to culture on artificial media.

204 Donovanosis — lesions. The disease is usually confined to the genitalia, but other sites may be affected. In men the penis is the common site, in women the labia. The primary lesion is an indurated nodule, which becomes ulcerated. Individual lesions may coalesce to form enlarging areas of ulceration, and autoinfection may occur. In this patient from Papua New Guinea spread of infection to the inguinal lymph nodes from the initial penile lesion has resulted in extensive ulceration in the groins. Secondary infection may cause further damage and scarring may lead to deformity.

203

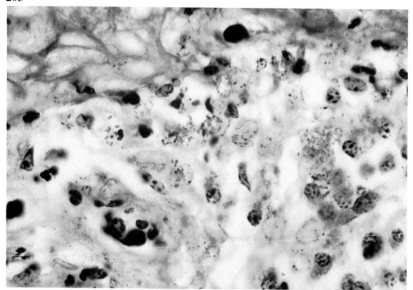

204

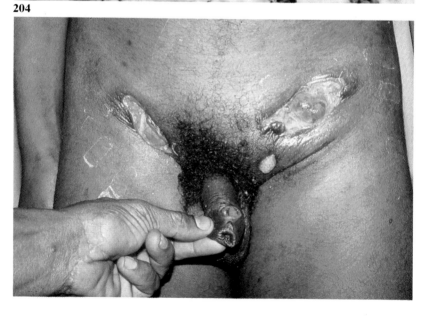

VIRUS INFECTIONS

Herpesvirus group

Members of this group cause important infections in both man and animals. Those associated with disease in man include:

- *Herpesvirus varicellae/zoster* — the cause of chickenpox and herpes zoster.

- Herpes simplex virus.

- *Herpesvirus simiae* — a rare cause of encephalitis in man.

- Cytomegalovirus — benign lymphadenitis and other syndromes.

- Epstein–Barr virus — associated with infectious mononucleosis and neoplastic disease.

The herpesviruses are relatively large, 120 to 180nm, with a central capsid containing DNA and an outer membrane derived from the host cell. They are ether-sensitive. They develop within the nucleus of the host cell and may pass quietly into the cytoplasm and leave the cell without necessarily destroying it. An acidophilic inclusion body surrounded by a halo (Cowdry type A) is characteristically left in the nucleus as a memorial to viral replication. Many viruses in the group show a marked tendency to latency and may become active whenever host immunity is impaired.

Varicella (chickenpox)

Varicella is a highly infectious disease mainly affecting young children, though no age group is exempt. Infection is usually acquired by direct contact with a case during the first few days of illness, when virus is being shed from the respiratory mucosa and skin. The virus is probably transmitted by the airborne route and enters through the respiratory passages. The incubation period varies but commonly lies between 15 and 18 days. In children varicella is generally mild and complications are rare; in adults the illness tends to be more severe with a higher incidence of complications.

The viruses causing chickenpox and herpes zoster appear to be identical and have been designated *Herpesvirus varicellae/zoster*.

Virology and pathology

205 **Electron micrograph of** *Herpesvirus varicellae/zoster.* On electron microscopy the viruses of varicella, herpes zoster, and herpes simplex are identical. The fully mature particle in the vesicular fluid measures about 150 to 200nm in diameter. There is an electron-dense inner core of DNA enclosed by a shell or capsid. This capsid has an icosahedral structure with an axial symmetry of 5:3:2, and consists of 162 capsomeres, which appear as hollow cylinders with a polygonal cross-section. The outer membrane of the virus is derived from the nuclear membrane of the host cell. Herpesviruses are easily distinguished from poxvirus by electron microscopy.

206 *Herpesvirus varicellae/zoster* **in human amnion cells.** Chickenpox virus does not grow on the chorioallantois of chick embryos, but can be propagated in a variety of primary cultures of human tissues and in some cultures of monkey tissues. In human amnion culture focal lesions appear in the cell sheet and spread slowly outwards as contiguous cells become infected. Typical intranuclear inclusion bodies are found in the degenerate cells. The supernatant fluid remains free from virus. Chickenpox virus grows readily in human thyroid cells and may be harvested from the supernatant fluid for neutralisation tests. (Arrow = cell with intranuclear inclusion.)

207 **Giant cell in human amnion cell culture.** Multinucleated giant cells are a characteristic feature in human tissues or in cultures of cells infected with chickenpox virus. The nuclei of these cells contain typical eosinophilic type A inclusions. (Arrow = nucleus with inclusion.)

205

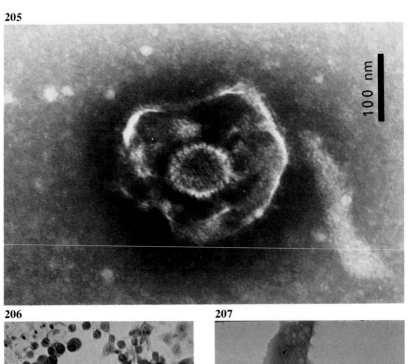

206 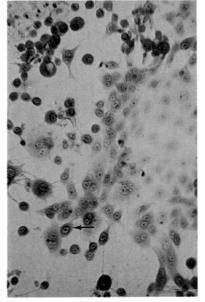 **207**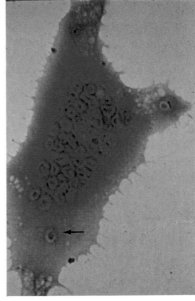

208   Histology of early chickenpox vesicle. The vesicles of varicella, zoster and herpes simplex cannot be distinguished from each other histologically, but may be differentiated from those of poxvirus infections and vaccinia by the presence of multinucleated giant cells.

Vesicles form within the epidermis as a result of cellular degeneration accompanied by intracellular oedema. At first the fluid collects in small pockets, but these eventually merge to form the mature vesicle.

Two types of degeneration are found — 'ballooning' and reticular. 'Ballooning' is peculiar to virus infections but reticular degeneration is also seen in some forms of dermatitis. In 'ballooning' degeneration the epidermal cells swell, lose their intercellular prickles, and become separated from each other. The cytoplasm is intensely eosinophilic. In reticular degeneration the cells swell but remain clear; some may eventually rupture. (A = intra-epidermal vesicle, B = multinucleated giant cell.)

209   Mature vesicle. The small foci seen in **208** have now coalesced to form a large vesicle. There is little cellular reaction in the dermis and the epithelial cells usually survive intact, so scarring seldom follows. An occasional polymorphonuclear cell may be present in the vesicular fluid. (A = intra-epidermal vesicle, B = dermis.)

Clinical features

210   Distribution of rash. A prodromal illness seldom occurs in children, but occasionally the exanthem in adults may be preceded by fever, headache, and sore throat.

Skin lesions are seen first on the body and inner aspects of the thighs but spread quickly to the face, scalp, and proximal parts of the limbs. The distribution of the rash used to be supremely important in differentiating varicella from variola. The rash in chickenpox is heaviest on the trunk and diminishes in intensity towards the periphery. It is prominent on flexor surfaces and extends into the hollows of the body.

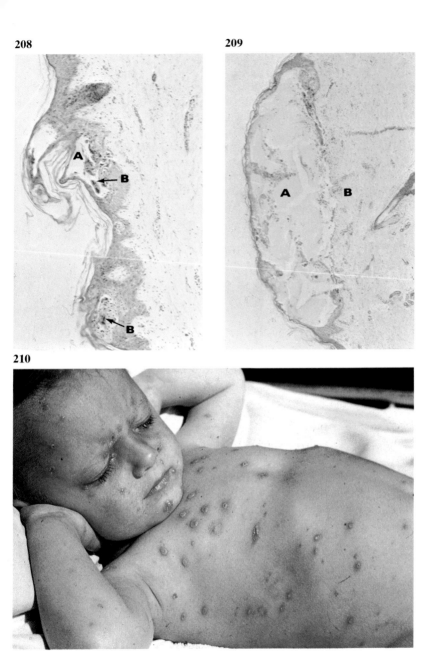

211   Chickenpox rash on dark skin. Detection of a chickenpox rash on heavily pigmented skin is easy: although the individual lesions may appear slightly different, the rash conforms to the rule of centripetal distribution. In this illustration the spots are dense on the arm but gradually diminish on the forearm to become scanty on the hand.

212   Pleomorphic rash. The rash evolves very rapidly through the stages of macule, papule, vesicle, pustule and crust. The first two stages are seldom seen, and the rash has usually reached the vesicular stage before it is discovered. Many lesions abort without undergoing full development.

In chickenpox the lesions emerge in crops at irregular intervals up to a week. As a result, the rash has a pleomorphic character with spots at different stages of development. Pruritus may be very troublesome during the first few days.

211

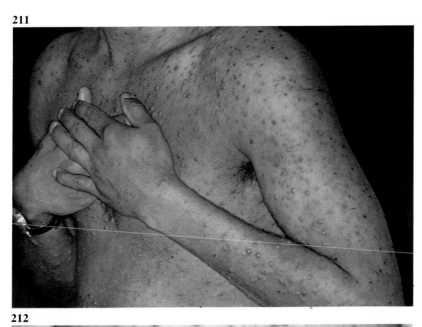

212

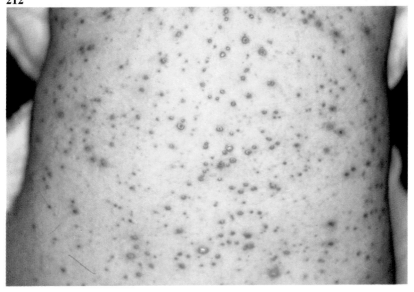

213   Close-up of rash on dark skin. In dark-skinned patients it is very common to find a petechial element in the rash and bleeding into the vesicles. The prognosis is not affected by these skin haemorrhages.

214   Close-up of lesions on white skin. Skin lesions vary greatly in size and shape. Fully developed vesicles and pustules are often oval but may be round or even totally irregular. The long axis of the oval lesion tends to follow the natural creases of the skin. Many lesions heal at an early stage. Skin haemorrhages are rare in white patients.

The chickenpox vesicle is unilocular and lies on the surface of the skin like a drop of water. When mature it is often surrounded by an erythematous ring or areola. After two or three days the vesicular fluid becomes cloudy, and a pustule forms with crenated edges.

215   Scarring. Most chickenpox lesions are very superficial, and damaged epidermis is quickly restored, leaving the skin unblemished. Occasionally the damage extends more deeply into the skin, and unsightly scarring results.

216   Close-up of scar. A pitted or foveated scar is the only clinical evidence that a patient has previously had chickenpox. Similar scars may be produced by vaccination against smallpox or by BCG immunisation.

213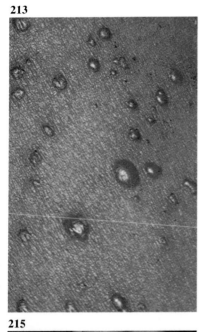

214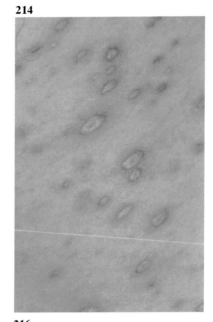

215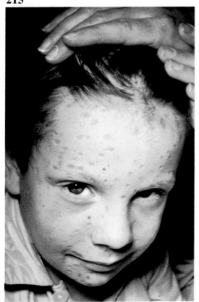

216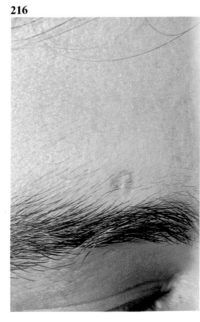

217 Petechiae on palate. Fine haemorrhages may be found on the palate in varicella as in many other infections. A vesicle is beginning to form on the palate above the left tonsil.

218 Vesicles on palate. During the first day or two the throat may be painful and inflamed, but no focal lesions are seen. Vesicles may later erupt on the palate and pharynx adding to the discomfort. The thin roof of the vesicle usually ruptures and leaves a shallow ulcer, which heals without scarring.

219 Vesicles on tongue. Vesicles may be found on the mucosa of the mouth and respiratory tract. On the tongue vesicles have a flat top and heal without forming a crust.

220 Vesicle on conjunctiva. Vesicles may be found on the conjunctivae where they pursue a benign course and heal without scarring.

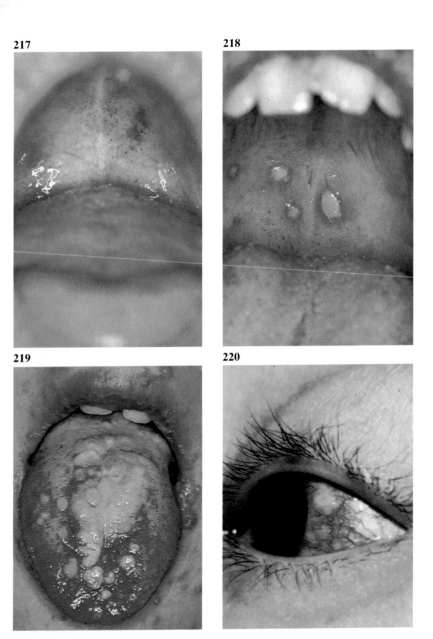

Complications

221   Varicella and bullous impetigo. Secondary infection of chickenpox lesions with *Staphylococcus aureus* may give rise to bullous impetigo with widespread infection of the surface of the skin.

222   Gangrene of skin. Invasion of the deeper layers of the skin and subcutaneous tissues by a virulent staphylococcus may result in cellulitis with gangrene and deep ulceration.

Septicaemia may develop with or without evidence of local sepsis, and blood cultures should be performed whenever a patient is unusually ill or the fever unduly prolonged.

223   Varicella and 'surgical' scarlet fever. Local infection of a chickenpox lesion by a haemolytic streptococcus in a patient susceptible to erythrogenic toxin may result in an attack of scarlet fever. The infected lesions can be identified by the surrounding inflammation. Toxin is absorbed from the skin and produces the generalised punctate erythema of scarlet fever.

224   Varicella and 'surgical' scarlet fever — tongue. Although the streptococcus is growing in the skin and not in the throat, the patient nevertheless develops a typical enanthem with a white strawberry tongue (see **27**).

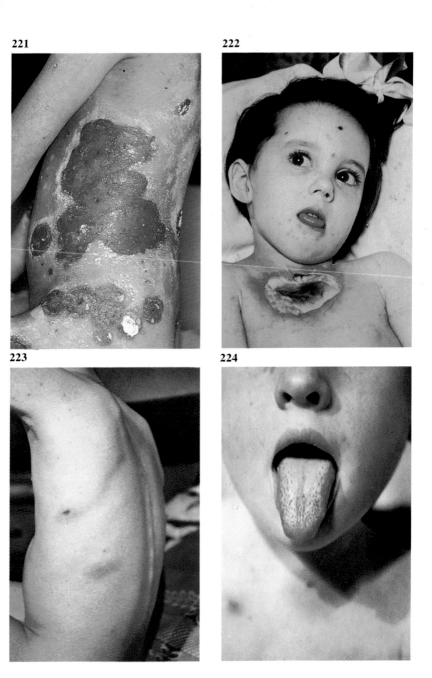

225 Chest x-ray of child with staphylococcal pyopneumothorax. Pneumonia complicating chickenpox in children is usually caused by secondary bacterial invasion from the upper respiratory passages, and is predominantly staphylococcal. Abscesses may form in the lungs.

This child's chest x-ray shows gross displacement of the mediastinum caused by pyopneumothorax, which resulted from rupture of a subpleural abscess. Each time the child coughed more air was forced into the pleural cavity through the pulmonary fistula, and continuous suction was necessary to reduce the pressure. Pus aspirated from the chest gave a heavy growth of *Staph. aureus*.

226 Chickenpox pneumonia. Chest x-ray — first week. Chickenpox viral pneumonia is found typically in adult patients and only very exceptionally in children. The condition varies greatly in severity: at one extreme it is so mild that it can be detected only by routine radiography; at the other it presents as a catastrophic illness with severe dyspnoea, cyanosis, haemoptysis and prostration, terminating fatally within 24 to 48 hours.

In a typical case the lungs are affected within two to five days from the onset of the rash. During the first week of the illness the characteristic findings are those of acute inflammatory pulmonary oedema. Dyspnoea and cyanosis are prominent. X-ray examination of the chest at this stage shows widespread soft nodular opacities throughout both lungs, but less noticeable at the apices.

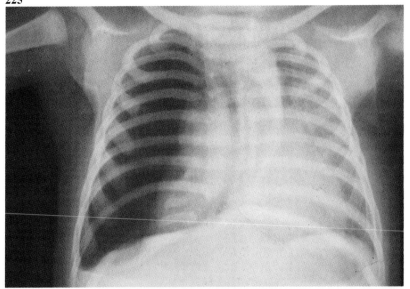

226

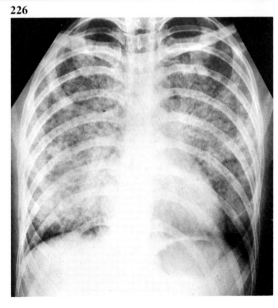

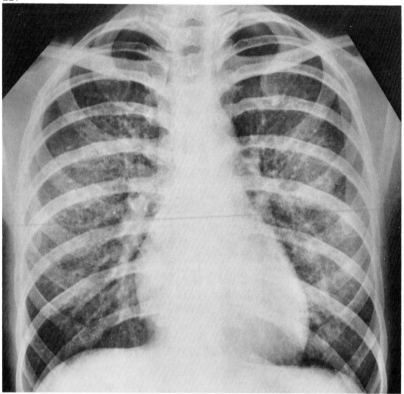

227 Chickenpox pneumonia. Chest x-ray — second week. Mortality is high in pregnant women and in patients with disturbed immunity, who commonly die from respiratory failure during the first week. During the second week the pulmonary oedema abates and the patient begins to improve. The cough lessens, and the abnormal chest signs disappear. Towards the end of the second week the chest radiograph shows changes, as the soft nodular shadowing resolves, leaving a prominent reticular pattern.

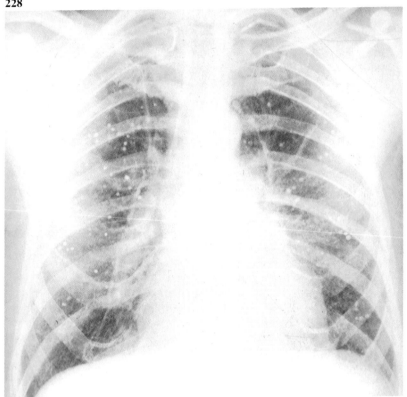

228   Chickenpox pneumonia. Chest x-ray — miliary calcification. After two weeks the patient emerges from the acute stage to face a prolonged period of convalescence. Breathlessness on slight exertion may persist for several weeks or even months, but eventually subsides, and full health is restored. In most patients the coarse reticular pattern gradually fades, though the chest radiograph may reveal abnormalities for many months. Patients found on routine examination to have miliary calcification of the lungs often give a history of severe chickenpox in adult life, and it is believed that calcium salts are deposited in the necrotic foci that are a typical feature of chickenpox pneumonia. Similar appearances may be found as a result of histoplasmosis or miliary tuberculosis.

229 Chickenpox pneumonia — histology of lung. In fatal cases of chickenpox pneumonia the lungs are grossly oedematous, and there are extensive haemorrhages. Histological examination shows widely disseminated interstitial pneumonia with patchy haemorrhagic consolidation.

The illustration shows a 3mm focus of fibrinoid necrosis surrounded by a zone of septal oedema and haemorrhage.

230 Chickenpox pneumonia — alveolar exudate. The alveoli are filled with a protein-rich fluid containing red cells and mononuclear cells. To the left of centre may be seen a degenerate mononuclear cell with a typical intranuclear inclusion. The nuclear membrane is clearly visible, but the cytoplasm is faintly stained. (Arrow = nuclear membrane with inclusion body.)

231 Haemorrhagic chickenpox. Widespread and sometimes fatal bleeding into the skin and mucous membranes may be precipitated by a number of infections, including chickenpox. The extent of the haemorrhages is not necessarily related to the severity of the original illness. In haemorrhagic chickenpox the platelet count is very low, the prothrombin time prolonged, and there may be other evidence of excessive consumption of clotting factors. Intravascular coagulation and endothelial damage by the virus may both contribute to the patient's death. Extensive haemorrhages into the skin or mucous membranes may be accompanied by alarming epistaxis, haematemesis, or haematuria.

232 Concurrent varicella and measles. The importance of the interference phenomenon varies with different virus infections. Sometimes infection with one virus may completely prevent invasion by another. This applies particularly to closely related viruses, such as members of the enterovirus group, but seldom occurs when viruses have notably different characteristics.

In the illustration a chickenpox rash is emerging on the upper limb of a child with a florid measles rash.

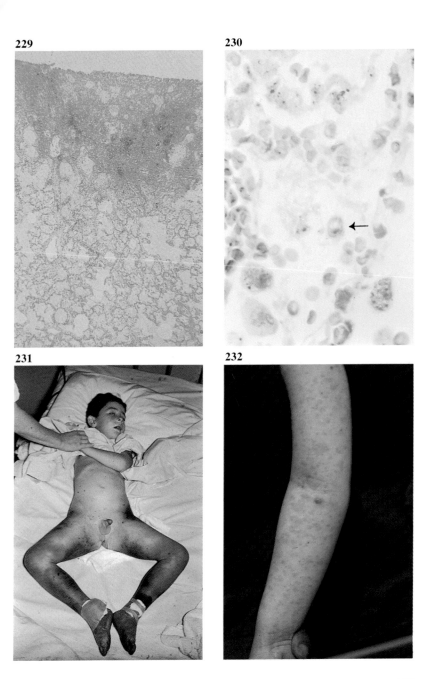

Varicella in disturbed immunity

233 Varicella and disturbed immunity. Patients with underlying disease affecting immunity are especially vulnerable to chickenpox, which may follow an exceptionally severe or prolonged course and may terminate in death.

The illustration shows a patient with Hodgkin's disease who contracted chickenpox from her child. Although the rash was not particularly dense, the individual lesions were unusually large and the general disturbance severe. Jaundice developed and 'cropping' continued until the patient died three or four weeks after the onset of her illness.

234 Close-up of lesions in chickenpox associated with defective immunity. The large size of the lesions is striking. The pustular fluid was sterile on culture for bacteria.

Patients who have never had chickenpox and who have defective immunity as a result of disease of the reticuloendothelial system or immunosuppressive treatment, are in grave danger from chickenpox and should not be exposed to this disease or to herpes zoster.

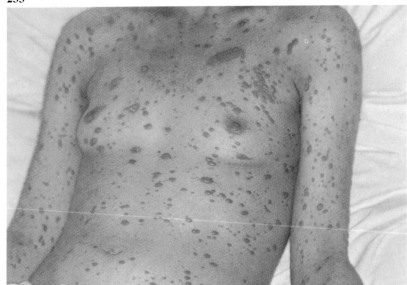

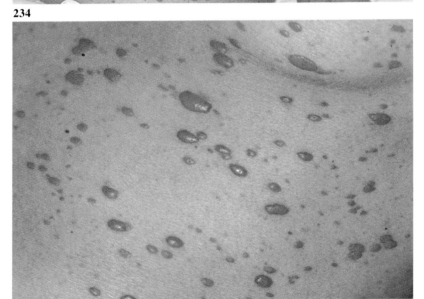

Herpes zoster (shingles)

Pathology

235 Histology of dorsal root ganglion. Herpes zoster is believed to be caused by reactivation of varicella virus lying dormant in cells of a dorsal root ganglion. In the early stages there is an acute inflammatory reaction in the ganglion, or its equivalent in the cranial nerves, which extends into the dorsal root and involves the meninges and spinal cord. Mononuclear cells are conspicuous, but there is a notable absence of polymorphonuclear cells. (A = undegenerate neurones, B = degenerate neurones, C = mononuclear cells.)

236 Histology of peripheral nerve. Virus spreads from the dorsal root ganglion cells along the sensory nerve fibres to the skin, where it enters the epithelial cells. At this stage virus particles may be found in the nuclei and cytoplasm of ganglion cells, in the cytoplasm of perineural cells, in the nuclei and cytoplasm of Schwann cells, and in the nuclei and cytoplasm of cells in the epidermis.

The illustration shows a section of frontal nerve from a patient with trigeminal herpes, who died four days after the onset of the rash. Staining by fluorescent antibody demonstrates viral antigen in two nerve fibre bundles with heavy concentration in the perineurium.

237 Histology of vesicle. The vesicles of herpes zoster and varicella are identical. The vesicle forms in the epidermis as a result of degeneration of the cells, which become swollen and separated, and some rupture. Intercellular oedema is marked and giant cells are a prominent feature. Severe inflammatory reaction in the corium may be followed by scarring.

In this section inflammatory reaction is slight, but many bizarre cells are present. (A = intra-epidermal vesicle, B = multinucleated giant cell, C = dermis.)

235

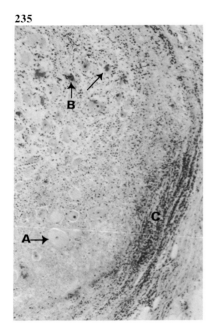

236

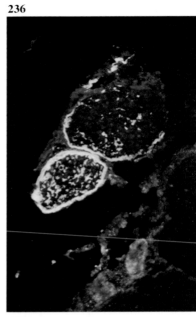

237

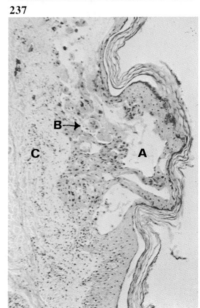

238 Effect of nerve damage on distribution of rash. A patient with hypoaesthesia, a result of section of a cutaneous nerve during a herniotomy 15 months previously, developed an attack of herpes zoster involving the same dermatome. Virus spread readily into the skin where sensation was normal, but round the scar, where the nerve supply had been interrupted, the skin was spared. This would be expected if the virus in herpes zoster gains access to the epidermis along nerve pathways.

Clinical features

239 Evolution of rash — erythema. An attack of herpes zoster begins with pain and hyperaesthesia in the distribution of one or two adjacent sensory nerve roots. Within a few days a rash appears in the same area. At first the skin has a deep red flush, but clusters of vesicles soon emerge. The rash is strictly confined to the midline, but oedema may spread extensively wherever subcutaneous tissues are lax.

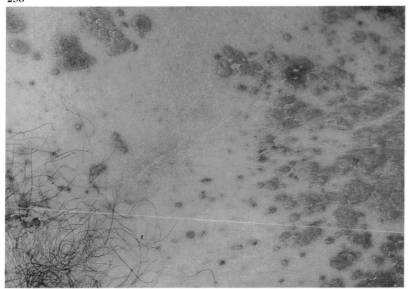

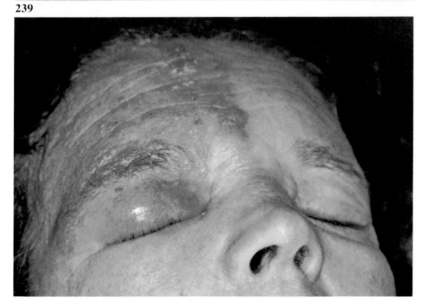

240 Evolution of rash — vesicles. The severity of the illness and extent of the rash are extremely variable. Fresh crops of vesicles continue to emerge for several days and may coalesce to form bullae, some of which may be haemorrhagic.

241 Evolution of rash — pustules. After a week or so the vesicles begin to dry up and form scabs but some may go through an intermediate pustular stage. These are usually sterile on bacterial culture.

242 Evolution of rash — crusts. If the rash is heavy, and especially if there is damage to the underlying corium, a thick plate of scabs may form which takes several weeks to separate. Any attempt at forcible removal merely results in the formation of fresh scabs and further harm to the skin. With a rash of average severity the scabs have usually been shed within two or three weeks.

240

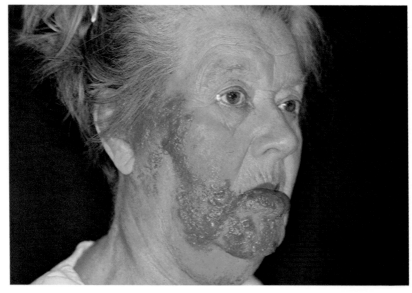

241

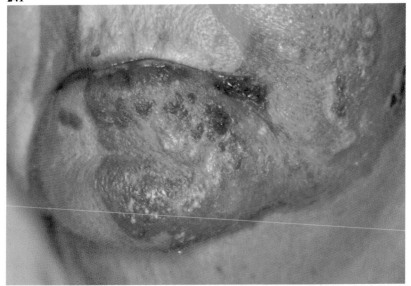

242

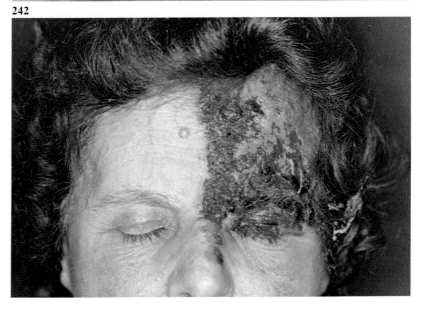

243 Evolution of rash — ulcers. In most attacks skin will heal without scars. Should the crusts separate and produce deep ulceration then scarring is inevitable. Heavy pigmentation may persist in the damaged area for many months.

244 Close-up of vesicles. The vesicles develop in clusters on an erythematous base.

245 Close-up of pustules. At a later stage the fluid in the blisters becomes turbid, and pustules are formed. This is not due to secondary bacterial invasion but to the activity of the virus itself. Adjacent lesions tend to run into each other, and already a central crust is appearing. Haemorrhage is common in severe attacks and produces bluish discoloration.

243

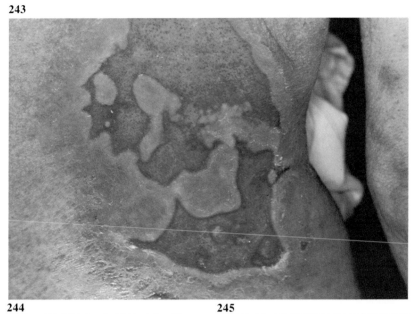

244

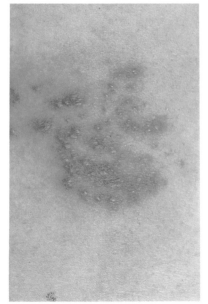

245

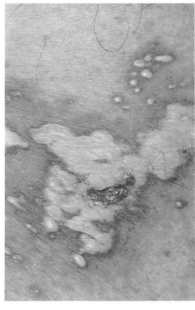

246 Distribution — cervical. The rash has sharply defined borders confined to the areas of skin supplied by cervical roots 4 and 5. This peculiar segmental distribution is a very helpful feature making it possible to distinguish herpes zoster from other similar rashes, particularly erysipelas (see **30**). Herpes simplex may simulate zoster, but pain is less troublesome, and the rash seldom conforms to a complete segmental distribution (see **284**).

247 Distribution — thoracic. Thoracic segments are affected in over 50% of patients with zoster. The rash is distributed in a band around the trunk. The term zoster is derived from the Greek meaning belt, and shingles from the Low Latin equivalent.

246

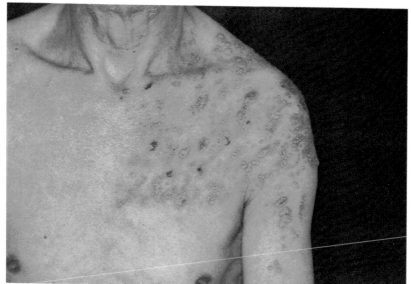

247

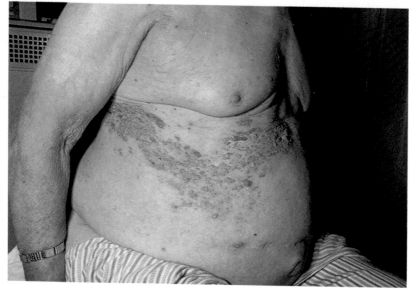

248   Distribution — thoracic. The rash seldom covers the entire area of skin in a dermatome. Lesions are grouped in clusters and generally form an unmistakeable pattern. The diagnosis may be difficult when the eruption consists of a single cluster, but a history of pain preceding the spots provides a helpful clue. In doubtful cases diagnosis can be established by demonstrating a rising antibody concentration in paired sera.

249   Herpes zoster with generalised rash. If patients with zoster are examined carefully, at least half will be found to have a sparse chickenpox rash. This emerges after the zoster, and the spots often abort at an early stage of development.

Moderate or heavy generalised varicella eruptions occur in 2 to 4% of cases, and are common when there is an underlying disturbance of immunity.

The standard sequence of events is reactivation of virus in the dorsal root ganglion with spread of virus along the sensory nerves to the skin segment, followed by dissemination into the blood stream resulting in a generalised rash.

250   Herpes zoster in a child. Herpes zoster is predominantly a disease of the middle-aged and elderly. Less than 5% of attacks occur in children below the age of 10 years. When zoster develops in very young children there is frequently a history of an attack of chickenpox in the mother during pregnancy. Post-herpetic neuralgia is seldom a problem in children.

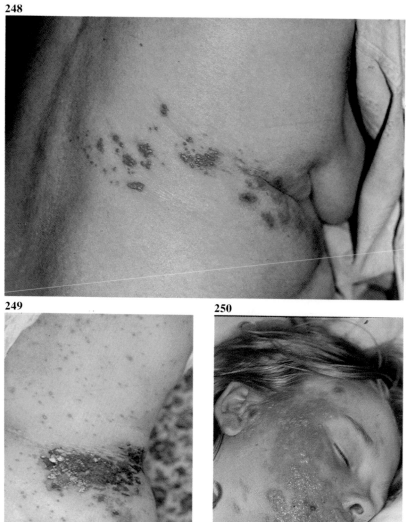

248

249

250

251 Herpes zoster of the palate. When an appropriate ganglion is affected lesions may be found on mucous membranes. Herpes zoster of the second division of the fifth cranial nerve affects the palate as well as the skin over the maxilla.

Complications

252 Conjunctivitis. Conjunctivitis may persist for several weeks after an attack of ophthalmic herpes, especially in the elderly, and may be associated with keratitis or iridocyclitis.

253 Corneal ulceration. During convalescence, after an attack of ophthalmic herpes, minor trauma to the anaesthetic cornea may abrade the surface and result in troublesome ulceration. Continual dabbing at the painful watering eye by an elderly confused patient may produce a penetrating ulcer that could perforate the anterior chamber. In these circumstances tarsorrhaphy may be required to protect the eye until the ulcer heals.

254 Chemosis. Unilateral ophthalmic herpes may be accompanied by oedema of the eyelids on both sides of the face and by striking oedema of the conjunctiva on the affected side (chemosis). When the eyelids are opened, the oedematous conjunctiva protrudes as a yellow gelatinous bag. The condition is not serious and resolves quickly.

251

252

253

254

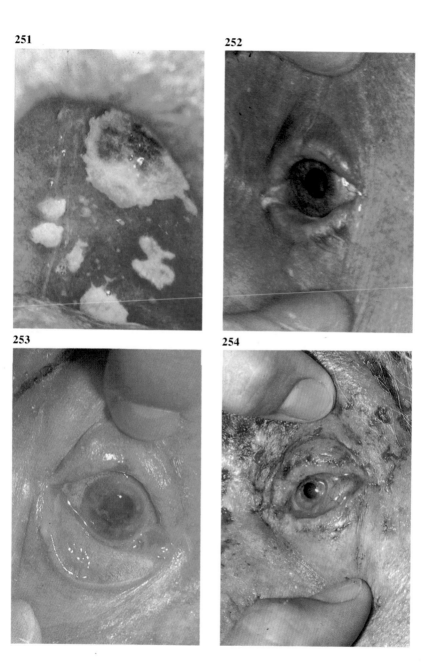

255 Iridocyclitis. The first division of the trigeminal nerve supplies the skin of the forehead and also the iris and ciliary body. A heavy rash on the side of the nose indicates that the nasociliary branch is severely affected, and iridocyclitis a strong probability.

The patient usually has difficulty in opening the oedematous eyelids so may not complain of defective vision. On examination the cornea is hazy and the pupil small. The reaction of the pupil is impaired, and the colour of the iris altered. When the pupil is dilated by a mydriatic the outline may be irregular as a result of adhesions between the iris and cornea.

256 Streptococcal impetigo. If herpetic lesions are kept dry, secondary bacterial infection is seldom a problem. Superimposed streptococcal infection may cause impetigo or erysipelas.

257 Secondary staphylococcal infection. A combination of zoster with a virulent staphylococcal infection may result in extensive damage to the corium and ugly scarring.

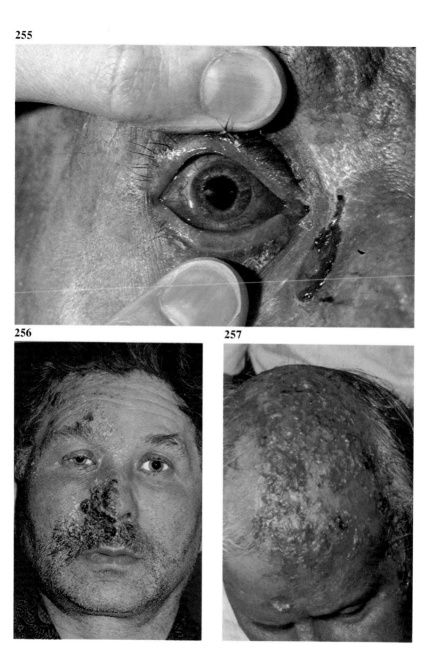

255

256

257

258 Herpes zoster with ophthalmoplegia. Spread of virus to lower motor neurone cells is not uncommon, and minor degrees of weakness are easily overlooked.

This patient had an attack of zoster involving the ophthalmic division of the fifth nerve complicated by ophthalmoplegia. He has ptosis and is unable to move his right eye. The conjunctiva is severely congested.

259 Facial paralysis complicating herpes zoster. Facial paralysis may follow herpes zoster of the trigeminal nerve, the geniculate ganglion of the seventh, or the second and third cervical roots. The exact pathways traversed by the virus are unknown.

This patient had zoster of the fifth cranial nerve, which resulted in facial weakness of lower motor neurone type and severe post-herpetic neuralgia.

258

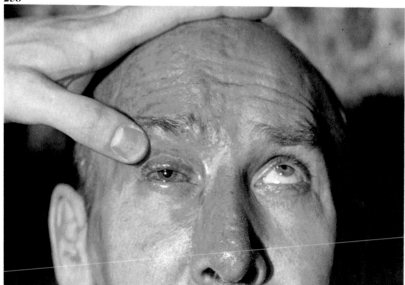

259

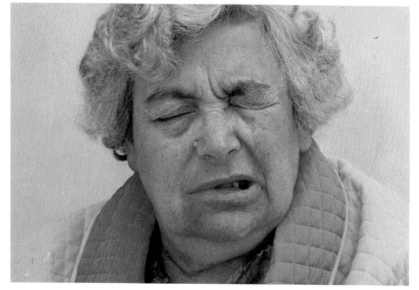

260 Geniculate herpes. Zoster of the geniculate ganglion of the seventh cranial nerve produces a crop of vesicles on the pinna and gives rise to facial paralysis accompanied by loss of taste over the anterior two-thirds of the tongue. Deafness may occur. The prognosis depends on the initial severity of the weakness.

261 Herpes zoster of C2 and C3 with facial paralysis. The patient has widespread zoster of the right side of her neck complicated by facial paralysis and deafness. She is unable to close her right eye, and her mouth is drawn over to the left. A year later the paralysis showed no improvement.

262 Herpes zoster of C4 and C5 with paralysis. During an attack of zoster affecting the fourth and fifth cervical roots, this elderly patient complained of 'rheumatism' in her right shoulder. Examination revealed that the stiffness was caused by weakness of the shoulder muscles. In attempting to abduct her arm the patient compensated for the deltoid paralysis by raising her shoulder and rotating her scapula.

260

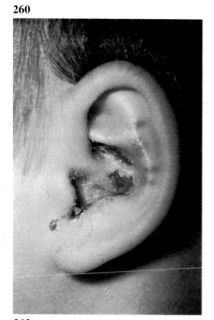

261

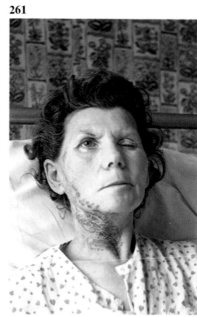

262

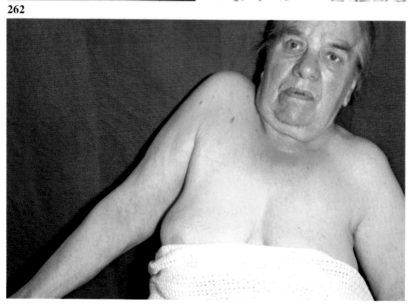

263 and 264 Horner's syndrome. The autonomic nervous system may also be affected by herpes zoster. This patient, with zoster of T2, developed Horner's syndrome on the affected side. Enophthalmos and a small pupil persisted for a few weeks then cleared.

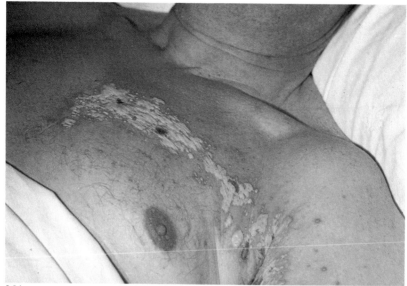

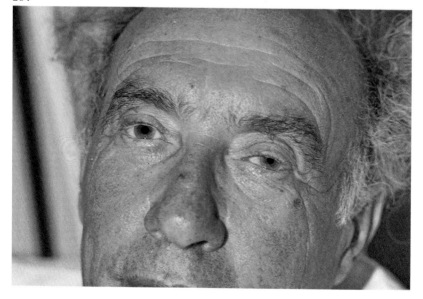

Associated diseases

265 Herpes zoster and leukaemia. An attack of herpes zoster may be precipitated by any condition that depresses immunity and allows the latent virus to emerge. All patients with zoster should be examined carefully for enlarged lymph nodes, splenomegaly, or hepatomegaly. The presence of undiagnosed lymphatic leukaemia may be signposted by an attack of shingles.

266 Herpes zoster and Hodgkin's disease. About 8% of patients admitted to hospital with zoster are found to have an underlying disease such as leukaemia, Hodgkin's disease, or carcinomatosis. Attacks may also be precipitated by immunosuppressive treatment. In such patients the skin lesions are often haemorrhagic and necrotic. The general disturbance is severe, and many patients die.

267 Herpes zoster and carcinomatosis. Metastases from surgically treated breast cancer were discovered when the patient developed a severe attack of herpes zoster and a heavy chickenpox rash. Many of the skin lesions are necrotic and the patient is jaundiced. The liver is enlarged and the abdomen distended by ascites. X-ray examination of the chest showed secondary deposits in the lungs.

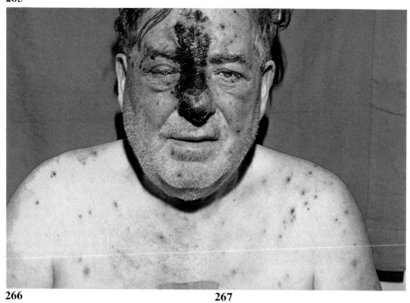

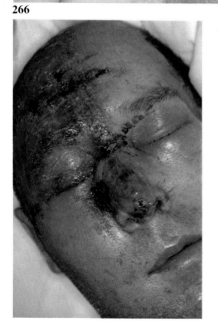

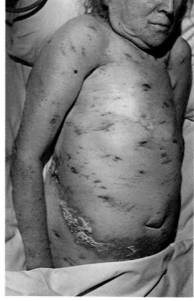

Herpes simplex infection

Primary infection with herpes simplex virus usually occurs in early childhood but may be deferred until adult life. In most children the reaction to the initial invasion is trivial with a few sores round the mouth, but a few develop acute gingivostomatitis and may be extremely ill. Subclinical infections are not uncommon. Once acquired, the virus may remain dormant for many years in cells of sensory nerve ganglia and has been detected in a high proportion of ganglia removed immediately after death.

Recurrent attacks are common and generally infect the skin around the mouth, although other sites may be affected. Herpes simplex virus is also responsible for infections of the central nervous system, eye and genital tract; it is suspected to be an etiological factor in squamous carcinoma of the lip and in carcinoma of the cervix of the uterus. Patients with eczema are especially susceptible to the virus and may succumb to generalised infection.

Herpes simplex virus of man is one of a large group of similar viruses naturally infecting many mammals and birds. Of these only B virus of monkeys is known to cause human disease. Herpes simplex virus can be separated into two types according to antigenic differences and biological characteristics. A small number of strains do not fall readily into either group.

Virology

268   Herpes simplex virus type 1 on chorioallantoic membrane. Type 1 viruses are usually isolated from the mouth or throat, from skin lesions, or from the brain of adults with encephalitis.

All human strains of the virus grow readily on chick embryo. Lesions appear on the chorioallantois within 24 to 28 hours after inoculation, and reach their maximum size in three to four days. The pocks produced by type 1 virus are smaller (less than 0.5 mm diameter) but more numerous than those produced by type 2. They are also more superficial.

269   Herpes simplex virus type 2 on chorioallantoic membrane. Type 2 viruses are usually isolated from the genital tract but may be recovered from brain and other organs in neonatal infection.

Fewer lesions are produced on chorioallantoic membrane by type 2 viruses but the lesions are large (more than 1 mm diameter) and more deeply seated.

268

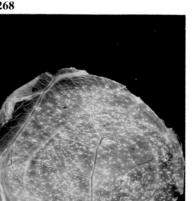

269

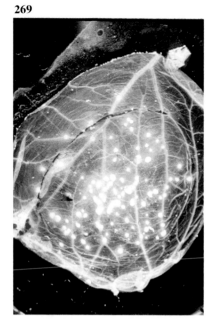

270 Normal monkey kidney cell culture.

271 Herpes simplex virus in monkey kidney cells. Chick embryo is no longer used for primary isolation of herpes simplex virus but is still used for confirming the type. Isolation of the virus is accomplished more easily in tissue cultures of primary rabbit kidney or primary human amnion cells, although many other cells are suitable. The growth of the virus can be recognised by cytopathogenic changes, which appear within 24 to 48 hours. These vary with the type of virus and the nature of the host cells. A lytic effect is produced in amnion cells and multinucleated giant cells may be found in HeLa cell cultures. In monkey kidney cell culture the infected cells degenerate and become rounded.

Clinical syndromes

272 Disseminated herpes infection in neonate. Focal necrosis of liver. Spread of infection from the mother's genital tract at birth or from an attendant may result in severe generalised infection culminating in death. Evidence of infection usually appears four to five days after birth. Local lesions may be found on the surface of the body but these are quickly overshadowed by the catastrophic general disturbance.

Foci of miliary necrosis are found in many organs and are particularly prominent in the liver. The condition may be mistaken for miliary tuberculosis. (Arrows = necrotic foci.)

273 Acute disseminated herpes — histology of liver. Intranuclear inclusion bodies are found in cells adjacent to areas of necrosis. When fully developed the inclusion is eosinophilic and Feulgen-negative. An unstained halo separates the inclusion from the nuclear membrane.

Around the edge of the lesion some of the cells show evidence of impending necrosis. These cells may be identified by their pyknotic nuclei.

Herpes simplex virus type 2 is found in 80% of neonates with disseminated infection. (A = intranuclear inclusion, B = pyknotic nucleus.)

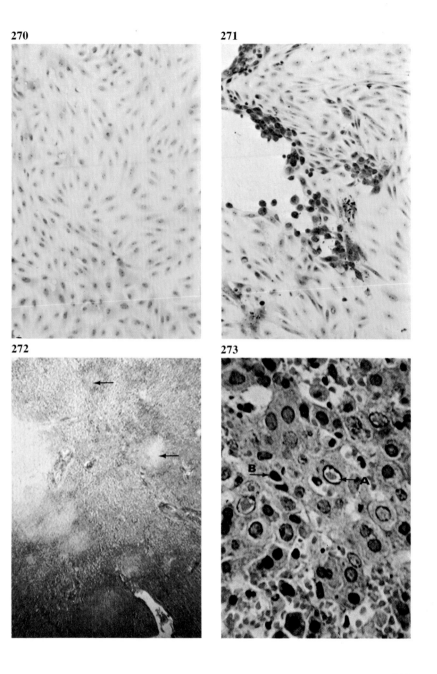

270

271

272

273

274 Herpetic encephalitis — section of brain. Infection of the central nervous system is more common than was previously thought. It may manifest as a meningo-encephalitis or encephalitis, generally associated with type 1 virus, or as aseptic meningitis, myelitis or radiculitis, generally associated with type 2 virus.

At autopsy there is intense engorgement of the brain and meninges with perivascular cuffing around the vessels in the cortex and subcortical white matter. The brain tissue is infiltrated with lymphocytes, plasma cells, and large mononuclear cells. Intranuclear inclusion bodies are found mainly in glial cells, but are also present in nerve cells.

Older children and adults may develop a localised form of encephalitis, mainly affecting the temporal lobe, which presents clinically as a space-occupying lesion. Necrosis is a striking feature of this localised form.

The section of brain shows perivascular cuffing with lymphocytes, plasma cells, and mononuclear cells. There are no polymorphonuclear cells or inclusions.

275 Neurones infected with herpes simplex virus. Fluorescent antibody staining shows viral antigens in nerve cells from a fatal case of herpetic encephalitis.

276 Acute disseminated herpes in older child — histology of liver. Fatal dissemination of the virus may occur in older children suffering from malnutrition. The changes in the tissues are similar to those found in neonatal infection. Type 1 virus is usually responsible.

This section of liver from an African child has been stained by fluorescent-antibody technique which indicates the presence of viral antigen along the portal tract.

274

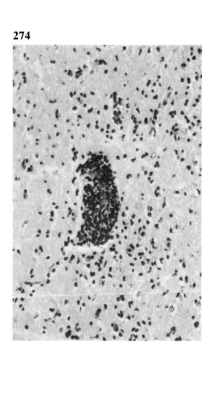

275

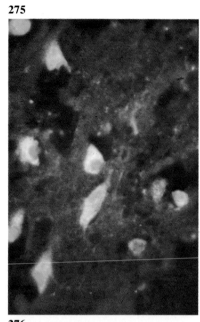

276

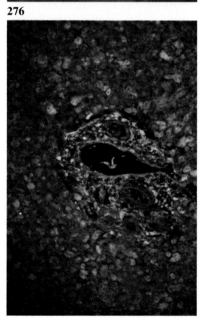

277 Histology of vesicle. At onset of infection cells in the deeper layers of the epidermis proliferate but degenerative changes soon follow. The affected cells swell, become separated from each other and some eventually rupture. Multinucleated giant cells may form. The underlying dermis is infiltrated by moderate numbers of neutrophil polymorphonuclear cells and lymphocytes.

The section is from hairy skin and shows a superficial vesicle that has destroyed the epidermis. The roof of the vesicle has collapsed and part of it may be seen at each side of the lesion. (A = edges of roof of vesicle, B = dermis, C = hair follicle, D = subcutaneous tissue.)

278 Primary gingivostomatitis in child. Herpes simplex virus is a very successful parasite and infection is widespread. In most communities about 60% of the population over five to six years old possess antibody against type 1 virus. Subclinical or mild infection is very common in early childhood, but primary infection in young children may occasionally provoke severe gingivostomatitis.

After a short prodromal illness lesions appear in the mouth. These consist of thin-walled vesicles on an erythematous base that soon rupture to form typical shallow ulcers with a serpiginous edge. The gums are particularly inflamed and swollen.

277

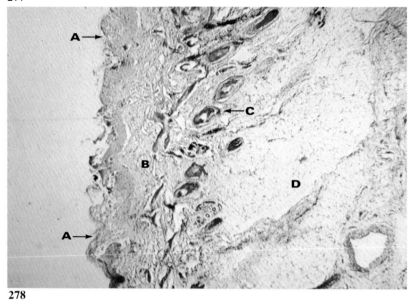

278

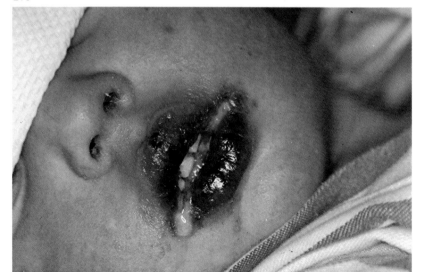

Notes

Notes

Notes

Notes

CIPRO®
(ciprofloxacin hydrochloride/Miles)
TABLETS

PZ100706

DESCRIPTION

Cipro* (ciprofloxacin hydrochloride) is a synthetic broad spectrum antibacterial agent for oral administration. Ciprofloxacin, a fluoroquinolone, is available as the monohydrochloride monohydrate salt of 1-cyclopropyl-6-fluoro-1, 4-dihydro-4-oxo-7-(1-piperazinyl)-3-quinolinecarboxylic acid. It is a faintly yellowish to light yellow crystalline substance with a molecular weight of 385.8. Its empirical formula is $C_{17}H_{18}FN_3O_3 \cdot HCl \cdot H_2O$ and its chemical structure is as follows:

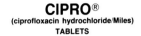

Cipro* is available in 250-mg, 500-mg and 750-mg (ciprofloxacin equivalent) film-coated tablets. The inactive ingredients are starch, microcrystalline cellulose, silicon dioxide, crospovidone, magnesium stearate, hydroxypropyl methylcellulose, titanium dioxide, polyethylene glycol and water. Ciprofloxacin differs from other quinolones in that it has a fluorine atom at the 6-position, a piperazine moiety at the 7-position, and a cyclopropyl ring at the 1-position. Examples of other antibacterial drugs in the quinolone class are nalidixic acid, cinoxacin, and norfloxacin.

CLINICAL PHARMACOLOGY

Cipro* tablets are rapidly and well absorbed from the gastrointestinal tract after oral administration. The absolute bioavailability is approximately 70% with no substantial loss by first pass metabolism. Serum concentrations increase proportionately with the dose as shown:

Dose (mg)	Maximum Serum Concentration (mcg/mL)	Area Under Curve (AUC) (mcg · hr/mL)
250	1.2	4.8
500	2.4	11.6
750	4.3	20.2
1000	5.4	30.8

Maximum serum concentrations are attained 1 to 2 hours after oral dosing. Mean concentrations 12 hours after dosing with 250, 500, or 750 mg are 0.1, 0.2, and 0.4 mcg/mL, respectively. The serum elimination half-life in subjects with normal renal function is approximately 4 hours.

Approximately 40 to 50% of an orally administered dose is excreted in the urine as unchanged drug. After a 250-mg oral dose, urine concentrations of ciprofloxacin usually exceed 200 mcg/mL during the first two hours and are approximately 30 mcg/mL at 8 to 12 hours after dosing. The urinary excretion of ciprofloxacin is virtually complete within 24 hours after dosing. The renal clearance of ciprofloxacin, which is approximately 300 mL/minute, exceeds the normal glomerular filtration rate of 120 mL/minute. Thus, active tubular secretion would seem to play a significant role in its elimination. Co-administration of probenecid with ciprofloxacin results in about a 50% reduction in the ciprofloxacin renal clearance and a 50% increase in its concentration in the systemic circulation. Although bile concentrations of ciprofloxacin are several fold higher than serum concentrations after oral dosing, only a small amount of the dose administered is recovered from the bile as unchanged drug. An additional 1-2% of the dose is recovered from the bile in the form of metabolites. Approximately 20 to 35% of an oral dose is recovered from the feces within 5 days after dosing. This may arise from either biliary clearance or transintestinal elimination. Four metabolites have been identified in human urine which together account for approximately 15% of an oral dose. The metabolites have antimicrobial activity, but are less active than unchanged ciprofloxacin.

When Cipro* is given concomitantly with food, there is a delay in the absorption of the drug, resulting in peak concentrations that are closer to 2 hours after dosing rather than 1 hour. The overall absorption, however, is not substantially affected. Concurrent administration of antacids containing magnesium hydroxide or aluminum hydroxide may reduce the bioavailability of ciprofloxacin by as much as 90% (See Precautions).

Concomitant administration of ciprofloxacin with theophylline decreases the clearance of theophylline resulting in elevated serum theophylline levels, and increased risk of a patient developing CNS or other adverse reactions (See Precautions).

In patients with reduced renal function, the half-life of ciprofloxacin is slightly prolonged. Dosage adjustments may be required (See Dosage and Administration).

In preliminary studies in patients with stable chronic liver cirrhosis, no significant changes in ciprofloxacin pharmacokinetics have been observed. The kinetics of ciprofloxacin in patients with acute hepatic insufficiency, however, have not been fully elucidated.

The binding of ciprofloxacin to serum proteins is 20 to 40% which is not likely to be high enough to cause significant protein binding interactions with other drugs.

After oral administration ciprofloxacin is widely distributed throughout the body. Tissue concentrations often exceed serum concentrations in both men and women, particularly in genital tissue including the prostate. Ciprofloxacin is present in active form in the saliva, nasal and bronchial secretions, sputum, skin blister fluid, lymph, peritoneal fluid, bile and prostatic secretions. Ciprofloxacin has also been detected in lung, skin, fat, muscle, cartilage, and bone. The drug diffuses into the cerebrospinal fluid (CSF); however, CSF concentrations are generally less than 10% of peak serum concentrations. Low levels of the drug have been detected in the aqueous and vitreous humors of the eye.

Microbiology: Ciprofloxacin has *in vitro* activity against a wide range of gram-negative and gram-positive organisms. The bactericidal action of ciprofloxacin results from interference with the enzyme DNA gyrase which is needed for the synthesis of bacterial DNA.

While *in vitro* studies have demonstrated the susceptibility of most strains of the following microorganisms, clinical efficacy for infections other than those included in the Indications and Usage Section has not been documented:

Gram-Negative: *Escherichia coli; Klebsiella pneumoniae; Klebsiella oxytoca; Enterobacter aerogenes; Enterobacter cloacae; Citrobacter diversus; Citrobacter freundii; Edwardsiella tarda; Salmonella enteritidis; Salmonella typhi; Shigella sonnei, Shigella flexneri; Proteus mirabilis; Proteus vulgaris; Providencia stuartii; Providencia rettgeri; Morganella morganii; Serratia marcescens; Yersinia enterocolitica; Pseudomonas aeruginosa; Acinetobacter calcoaceticus* subsp. *lwoffi; Acinetobacter calcoaceticus* subsp. *anitratus; Haemophilus influenzae; Haemophilus parainfluenzae; Haemophilus ducreyi; Neisseria gonorrhoeae; Neisseria meningitidis; Moraxella (Branhamella) catarrhalis; Campylobacter jejuni; Campylobacter coli; Aeromonas hydrophila; Aeromonas caviae; Vibrio cholerae; Vibrio parahaemolyticus; Vibrio vulnificus; Brucella melitensis; Pasteurella multocida; Legionella pneumophila.*

Gram-Positive: *Staphylococcus aureus* (including methicillin-susceptible and methicillin-resistant strains); *Staphylococcus epidermidis; Staphylococcus haemolyticus; Staphylococcus hominis; Staphylococcus saprophyticus; Streptococcus pyogenes; Streptococcus pneumoniae.*

Most strains of streptococci including *Streptococcus faecalis* are only moderately susceptible to ciprofloxacin as are *Mycobacterium tuberculosis* and *Chlamydia trachomatis.*

Most strains of *Pseudomonas cepacia* and some strains of *Pseudomonas maltophilia* are resistant to ciprofloxacin as are most anaerobic bacteria, including *Bacteroides fragilis* and *Clostridium difficile.*

Ciprofloxacin is slightly less active when tested at acidic pH. The inoculum size has little effect when tested *in vitro.* The minimum bactericidal concentration (MBC) generally does not exceed the minimum inhibitory concentration (MIC) by more than a factor of 2. Resistance to ciprofloxacin *in vitro* develops slowly (multiple-step mutation). Rapid one-step development of resistance has not been observed.

Ciprofloxacin does not cross-react with other antimicrobial agents such as beta-lactams or aminoglycosides; therefore, organisms resistant to these drugs may be susceptible to ciprofloxacin.

In vitro studies have shown that additive activity often results when ciprofloxacin is combined with other antimicrobial agents such as beta-lactams, aminoglycosides, clindamycin, or metronidazole; antagonism is observed only rarely.

Susceptibility Tests

Diffusion Techniques: Quantitative methods that require measurement of zone diameters give the most precise estimates of antibiotic susceptibility. One such procedure recommended for use with the 5-mcg ciprofloxacin disk is the National Committee for Clinical Laboratory Standards (NCCLS) approved procedure. Only a 5-mcg ciprofloxacin disk should be used, and it should not be used for testing susceptibility to less active quinolones; there are no suitable surrogate disks.

Results of laboratory tests using 5-mcg ciprofloxacin disks should be interpreted using the following criteria:

Zone Diameter (mm)	Interpretation
≥ 21	(S) Susceptible
16 – 20	(I) Intermediate (Moderately Susceptible)
≤ 15	(R) Resistant

Dilution Techniques: Broth and agar dilution methods, such as those recommended by the NCCLS, may be used to determine the minimum inhibitory concentration (MIC) of ciprofloxacin. MIC test results should be interpreted according to the following criteria:

MIC (mcg/mL)	Interpretation
≤ 1	(S) Susceptible
> 1 – ≤ 2	(I) Intermediate (Moderately Susceptible)
> 2	(R) Resistant

For any susceptibility test, a report of "susceptible" indicates that the pathogen is likely to respond to ciprofloxacin therapy. A report of "resistant" indicates that the pathogen is not likely to respond. A report of "intermediate" (moderately susceptible) indicates that the pathogen is expected to be susceptible to ciprofloxacin if high doses are used, or if the infection is confined to tissues and fluids in which high ciprofloxacin levels are obtained.

The Quality Control strains should have the following assigned daily ranges for ciprofloxacin.

QC Strains	Disk Zone Diameter (mm)	MIC (mcg/mL)
S. aureus (ATCC 25923)	22 – 30	
S. aureus (ATCC 29213)		0.25–1.0
E. coli (ATCC 25922)	30 – 40	0.008–0.03
P. aeruginosa (ATCC 27853)	25 – 33	0.25–1.0

INDICATIONS AND USAGE

Cipro® is indicated for the treatment of infections caused by susceptible strains of the designated microorganisms in the conditions listed below:

Lower Respiratory Infections caused by *Escherichia coli, Klebsiella pneumoniae, Enterobacter cloacae, Proteus mirabilis, Pseudomonas aeruginosa, Haemophilus influenzae, Haemophilus parainfluenzae,* and *Streptococcus pneumoniae.*

Skin and Skin Structure Infections caused by *Escherichia coli, Klebsiella pneumoniae, Enterobacter cloacae, Proteus mirabilis, Proteus vulgaris, Providencia stuartii, Morganella morganii, Citrobacter freundii, Pseudomonas aeruginosa, Staphylococcus aureus, Staphylococcus epidermidis,* and *Streptococcus pyogenes.*

Bone and Joint Infections caused by *Enterobacter cloacae, Serratia marcescens,* and *Pseudomonas aeruginosa.*

Urinary Tract Infections caused by *Escherichia coli, Klebsiella pneumoniae, Enterobacter cloacae, Serratia marcescens, Proteus mirabilis, Providencia rettgeri, Morganella morganii, Citrobacter diversus, Citrobacter freundii, Pseudomonas aeruginosa, Staphylococcus epidermidis,* and *Streptococcus faecalis.*

Infectious Diarrhea caused by *Escherichia coli* (enterotoxigenic strains), *Campylobacter jejuni*, *Shigella flexneri** and *Shigella sonnei** when antibacterial therapy is indicated.

*Efficacy for this organism in this organ system was studied in fewer than 10 infections.

Appropriate culture and susceptibility tests should be performed before treatment in order to isolate and identify organisms causing infection and to determine their susceptibility to ciprofloxacin. Therapy with Cipro® may be initiated before results of these tests are known; once results become available appropriate therapy should be continued. As with other drugs, some strains of *Pseudomonas aeruginosa* may develop resistance fairly rapidly during treatment with ciprofloxacin. Culture and susceptibility testing performed periodically during therapy will provide information not only on the therapeutic effect of the antimicrobial agent but also on the possible emergence of bacterial resistance.

CONTRAINDICATIONS

A history of hypersensitivity to ciprofloxacin is a contraindication to its use. A history of hypersensitivity to other quinolones may also contraindicate the use of ciprofloxacin.

WARNINGS

CIPROFLOXACIN SHOULD NOT BE USED IN CHILDREN, ADOLESCENTS, OR PREGNANT WOMEN. The oral administration of ciprofloxacin caused lameness in immature dogs. Histopathological examination of the weight-bearing joints of these dogs revealed permanent lesions of the cartilage. Related drugs such as nalidixic acid, cinoxacin and norfloxacin also produced erosions of cartilage of weight-bearing joints and other signs of arthropathy in immature animals of various species (See Animal Pharmacology).

PRECAUTIONS

General: As with other quinolones, ciprofloxacin may cause central nervous system (CNS) stimulation which may lead to tremor, restlessness, lightheadedness, confusion, and rarely to hallucinations or convulsive seizures. Therefore, ciprofloxacin should be used with caution in patients with known or suspected CNS disorders, such as severe cerebral arteriosclerosis or epilepsy, or other factors which predispose to seizures (See Adverse Reactions).

Anaphylactic reactions following the first dose, have been reported in patients receiving therapy with quinolones. Some reactions were accompanied by cardiovascular collapse, loss of consciousness, tingling, pharyngeal or facial edema, dyspnea, urticaria, and itching. Only a few patients had a history of hypersensitivity reaction. Anaphylactic reactions may require epinephrine and other emergency measures.Ciprofloxacin should be discontinued at the first sign of hypersensitivity or allergy.

Severe hypersensitivity reactions characterized by rash, fever, eosinophilia, jaundice, and hepatic necrosis with fatal outcome have been reported rarely (less than one per million prescriptions) in patients receiving ciprofloxacin along with other drugs. The possibility that these reactions were related to ciprofloxacin cannot be excluded. Ciprofloxacin should be discontinued at the first appearance of a skin rash or any sign of other hypersensitivity reaction.

Crystals of ciprofloxacin have been observed rarely in the urine of human subjects but more frequently in the urine of laboratory animals (See Animal Pharmacology). Crystalluria related to ciprofloxacin has been reported only rarely in man because human urine is usually acidic. Patients receiving ciprofloxacin should be well hydrated and alkalinity of the urine should be avoided. The recommended daily dose should not be exceeded.

Alteration of the dosage regimen is necessary for patients with impairment of renal function (See Dosage and Administration).

As with any potent drug, periodic assessment of organ system functions, including renal, hepatic, and hematopoietic function, is advisable during prolonged therapy.

Drug Interactions: As with other quinolones concurrent administration of ciprofloxacin with theophylline may lead to elevated plasma concentrations of theophylline and prolongation of its elimination half-life. This may result in increased risk of theophylline-related adverse reactions. If concomitant use cannot be avoided, plasma levels of theophylline should be monitored and dosage adjustments made as appropriate.

Quinolones, including ciprofloxacin, have also been shown to interfere with the metabolism of caffeine. This may lead to reduced clearance of caffeine and a prolongation of its plasma half life.

Antacids containing magnesium hydroxide or aluminum hydroxide, may interfere with the absorption of ciprofloxacin resulting in serum and urine levels lower than desired; concurrent administration of these agents with ciprofloxacin should be avoided.

Concomitant administration of the nonsteroidal anti-inflammatory drug fenbufen with a quinolone has been reported to increase the risk of CNS stimulation and convulsive seizures.

Probenecid interferes with renal tubular secretion of ciprofloxacin and produces an increase in the level of ciprofloxacin in the serum. This should be considered if patients are receiving both drugs concomitantly.

As with other broad spectrum antimicrobial agents, prolonged use of ciprofloxacin may result in overgrowth of non-susceptible organisms. Repeated evaluation of the patient's condition and microbial susceptibility testing is essential. If superinfection occurs during therapy, appropriate measures should be taken.

Information for Patients: Patients should be advised that ciprofloxacin may be taken with or without meals. The preferred time of dosing is two hours after a meal. Patients should also be advised to drink fluids liberally and not take antacids containing magnesium or aluminum.

Patients should be advised that ciprofloxacin may be associated with hypersensitivity reactions, even following a single dose, and to discontinue the drug at the first sign of a skin rash or other allergic reaction.

Ciprofloxacin may cause dizziness and lightheadedness; therefore patients should know how they react to this drug before they operate an automobile or machinery or engage in activities requiring mental alertness or coordination.

Patients should be advised that ciprofloxacin may increase the effects of theophylline and caffeine.

Carcinogenesis, Mutagenesis, Impairment of Fertility: Eight *in vitro* mutagenicity tests have been conducted with ciprofloxacin and the test results are listed below:

> Salmonella/Microsome Test (Negative)
> *E. coli* DNA Repair Assay (Negative)
> Mouse Lymphoma Cell Forward Mutation Assay (Positive)
> Chinese Hamster V_{79} Cell HGPRT Test (Negative)
> Syrian Hamster Embryo Cell Transformation Assay (Negative)
> *Saccharomyces cerevisiae* Point Mutation Assay (Negative)
> *Saccharomyces cerevisiae* Mitotic Crossover and Gene Conversion Assay (Negative)
> Rat Hepatocyte DNA Repair Assay (Positive)

Thus 2 of the 8 tests were positive but results of the following 3 *in vivo* test systems gave negative results:

> Rat Hepatocyte DNA Repair Assay
> Micronucleus Test (Mice)
> Dominant Lethal Test (Mice)

Long term carcinogenicity studies in mice and rats have been completed. After daily oral dosing for up to 2 years, there is no evidence that ciprofloxacin had any carcinogenic or tumorigenic effects in these species.

Pregnancy — Pregnancy Category C: Reproduction studies have been performed in rats and mice at doses up to 6 times the usual daily human dose and have revealed no evidence of impaired fertility or harm to the fetus due to ciprofloxacin. In rabbits, as with most antimicrobial agents, ciprofloxacin (30 and 100 mg/kg orally) produced gastrointestinal disturbances resulting in maternal weight loss and an increased incidence of abortion. No teratogenicity was observed at either dose. After intravenous administration, at doses up to 20 mg/kg, no maternal toxicity was produced and no embryotoxicity or teratogenicity was observed. There are, however, no adequate and well-controlled studies in pregnant women. SINCE CIPROFLOXACIN, LIKE OTHER DRUGS IN ITS CLASS, CAUSES ARTHROPATHY IN IMMATURE ANIMALS, IT SHOULD NOT BE USED IN PREGNANT WOMEN (See Warnings).

Nursing Mothers: It is not known whether ciprofloxacin is excreted in human milk; however, it is known that ciprofloxacin is excreted in the milk of lactating rats and that other drugs of this class are excreted in human milk. Because of this and because of the potential for serious adverse reactions from ciprofloxacin in nursing infants, a decision should be made to discontinue nursing or to discontinue the drug, taking into account the importance of the drug to the mother.

Pediatric Use: Patients under the age of 18 were not included in the clinical trials of ciprofloxacin because ciprofloxacin as well as other quinolones causes arthropathy in immature animals. Ciprofloxacin should not be used in children or adolescents (See Warnings).

ADVERSE REACTIONS

Ciprofloxacin is generally well-tolerated. During clinical investigation, 2,799 patients received 2,868 courses of the drug. Adverse events that were considered likely to be drug related occurred in 7.3% of courses, possibly related in 9.2%, and remotely related in 3.0%. Ciprofloxacin was discontinued because of an adverse event in 3.5% of courses, primarily involving the gastrointestinal system (1.5%), skin (0.6%), and central nervous system (0.4%). Those events typical of quinolones are italicized.

The most frequently reported events, drug related or not, were *nausea* (5.2%), *diarrhea* (2.3%), *vomiting* (2.0%), *abdominal pain/discomfort* (1.7%), *headache* (1.2%), *restlessness* (1.1%), and *rash* (1.1%).

Additional events that occurred in less than 1% of ciprofloxacin courses are listed below.

GASTROINTESTINAL: *(See above)*, painful oral mucosa, oral candidiasis, dysphagia, intestinal perforation, gastrointestinal bleeding.

CENTRAL NERVOUS SYSTEM: *(See above)*, *dizziness, lightheadedness, insomnia, nightmares, hallucinations, manic reaction, irritability, tremor, ataxia, convulsive seizures, lethargy, drowsiness, weakness, malaise, anorexia, phobia, depersonalization, depression, paresthesia.*

SKIN/HYPERSENSITIVITY: *(See above)*, *pruritus, urticaria, photosensitivity, flushing, fever, chills, angioedema, edema of the face, neck, lips, conjunctivae or hands;* cutaneous candidiasis, hyperpigmentation, erythema nodosum.
Allergic reactions ranging from urticaria to anaphylactic reactions have been reported (See Precautions).

SPECIAL SENSES: *blurred vision, disturbed vision (change in color perception, overbrightness of lights), decreased visual acuity, diplopia, eye pain, tinnitus, hearing loss, bad taste.*

MUSCULOSKELETAL: *joint or back pain, joint stiffness*, achiness, neck or chest pain, flare up of gout.

RENAL/UROGENITAL: *interstitial nephritis, nephritis, renal failure*, polyuria, urinary retention, urethral bleeding, vaginitis, acidosis.

CARDIOVASCULAR: palpitations, atrial flutter, ventricular ectopy, syncope, hypertension, angina pectoris, myocardial infarction, cardiopulmonary arrest, cerebral thrombosis.

RESPIRATORY: epistaxis, laryngeal or pulmonary edema, hiccough, hemoptysis, dyspnea, bronchospasm, pulmonary embolism.
Most of the adverse events reported were described as only mild or moderate in severity, abated soon after the drug was discontinued, and required no treatment.

In several instances nausea, vomiting, tremor, restlessness, agitation or palpitations were judged by investigators to be related to elevated plasma levels of theophylline possibly as a result of drug interaction with ciprofloxacin.

Other adverse events reported in the postmarketing phase include anaphylactoid reactions, Stevens-Johnson syndrome, exfoliative dermatitis, toxic epidermal necrolysis, hepatic necrosis, postural hypotension, possible exacerbation of myasthenia gravis, confusion, dysphasia, nystagmus, pseudomembranous colitis, dyspepsia, flatulence, and constipation. Also reported were agranulocytosis; elevation of serum triglycerides, serum cholesterol, blood glucose, serum potassium; prolongation of prothrombin time; albuminuria; candiduria, vaginal candidiasis; and renal calculi (See Precautions).

Adverse Laboratory Changes: Changes in laboratory parameters listed as adverse events without regard to drug relationship:

Hepatic   — Elevations of: ALT (SGPT) (1.9%), AST (SGOT) (1.7%), Alkaline Phosphatase (0.8%), LDH (0.4%), serum bilirubin (0.3%). Cholestatic jaundice has been reported.

Hematologic — Eosinophilia (0.6%), leukopenia (0.4%), decreased blood platelets (0.1%), elevated blood platelets (0.1%), pancytopenia (0.1%).

Renal   — Elevations of: Serum creatinine (1.1%), BUN (0.9%).

CRYSTALLURIA, CYLINDRURIA AND HEMATURIA HAVE BEEN REPORTED.

Other changes occurring in less than 0.1% of courses were: Elevation of serum gammaglutamyl transferase, elevation of serum amylase, reduction in blood glucose, elevated uric acid, decrease in hemoglobin, anemia, bleeding diathesis, increase in blood monocytes, leukocytosis.

OVERDOSAGE

Information on overdosage in humans is not available. In the event of acute overdosage the stomach should be emptied by inducing vomiting or by gastric lavage. The patient should be carefully observed and given supportive treatment. Adequate hydration must be maintained. Only a small amount of ciprofloxacin (<10%) is removed from the body after hemodialysis or peritoneal dialysis.

DOSAGE AND ADMINISTRATION

The usual adult dosage for patients with urinary tract infections is 250 mg every 12 hours. For patients with complicated infections caused by organisms not highly susceptible, 500 mg may be administered every 12 hours.

Lower respiratory tract infections, skin and skin structure infections, and bone and joint infections may be treated with 500 mg every 12 hours. For more severe or complicated infections, a dosage of 750 mg may be given every 12 hours.

The recommended dosage for Infectious Diarrhea is 500 mg every 12 hours.

DOSAGE GUIDELINES

Location of Infection	Type or Severity	Unit Dose	Frequency	Daily Dose
Urinary tract	Mild/Moderate	250 mg	q 12 h	500 mg
	Severe/Complicated	500 mg	q 12 h	1000 mg
Lower respiratory tract; Bone and Joint; Skin or Skin Structure	Mild/Moderate	500 mg	q 12 h	1000 mg
	Severe/Complicated	750 mg	q 12 h	1500 mg
Infectious Diarrhea	Mild/Moderate/Severe	500 mg	q 12 h	1000 mg

The determination of dosage for any particular patient must take into consideration the severity and nature of the infection, the susceptibility of the causative organism, the integrity of the patient's host-defense mechanisms, and the status of renal function.

The duration of treatment depends upon the severity of infection. Generally ciprofloxacin should be continued for at least 2 days after the signs and symptoms of infection have disappeared. The usual duration is 7 to 14 days; however, for severe and complicated infections more prolonged therapy may be required. Bone and joint infections may require treatment for 4 to 6 weeks or longer. Infectious Diarrhea may be treated for 5-7 days.

Impaired Renal Function: Ciprofloxacin is eliminated primarily by renal excretion; however, the drug is also metabolized and partially cleared through the biliary system of the liver and through the intestine. These alternate pathways of drug elimination appear to compensate for the reduced renal excretion in patients with renal impairment. Nonetheless, some modification of dosage is recommended, particularly for patients with severe renal dysfunction. The following table provides dosage guidelines for use in patients with renal impairment; however, monitoring of serum drug levels provides the most reliable basis for dosage adjustment:

RECOMMENDED STARTING AND MAINTENANCE DOSES
FOR PATIENTS WITH IMPAIRED RENAL FUNCTION

Creatinine Clearance (mL/min)	Dose
> 50	See Usual Dosage
30 – 50	250 – 500 mg q 12 h
5 – 29	250 – 500 mg q 18 h
Patients on hemodialysis or Peritoneal dialysis	250 – 500 mg q 24 h (after dialysis)

When only the serum creatinine concentration is known, the following formula may be used to estimate creatinine clearance.

$$\text{Men: Creatinine clearance (mL/min)} = \frac{\text{Weight (kg)} \times (140 - \text{age})}{72 \times \text{serum creatinine (mg/dL)}}$$

Women: 0.85 × the value calculated for men.

The serum creatinine should represent a steady state of renal function.

In patients with severe infections and severe renal impairment, a unit dose of 750 mg may be administered at the intervals noted above; however, patients should be carefully monitored and the serum ciprofloxacin concentration should be measured periodically. Peak concentrations (1-2 hours after dosing) should generally range from 2 to 4 mcg/mL.

For patients with changing renal function or for patients with renal impairment and hepatic insufficiency, measurement of serum concentrations of ciprofloxacin will provide additional guidance for adjusting dosage.

HOW SUPPLIED

Cipro* (ciprofloxacin hydrochloride) is available as round, slightly yellowish film-coated tablets containing 250 mg ciprofloxacin. The 250-mg tablet is coded with the word "Miles" on one side and "512" on the reverse side. Cipro* is also available as capsule shaped, slightly yellowish film-coated tablets containing 500 mg or 750 mg ciprofloxacin. The 500-mg tablet is coded with the word "Miles" on one side and "513" on the reverse side; the 750-mg tablet is coded with the word "Miles" on one side and "514" on the reverse side. Each tablet strength is available in bottles of 50's and in Unit Dose packages of 100.